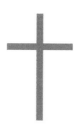

A Christian Diet

S. H. SHEPHERD

A Christian Diet

Scripture verses are mainly taken from the NKJV of the Holy Bible. Other translations used are the KJV, RSV, NIV and NLT.

"Have you not known?
Have you not heard?
Has it not been told you from the beginning?
Have you not understood from the foundations
of the earth?" - Isaiah 40:21.

To my mother, who taught me much about foods and nutrition, and who encouraged me to read the Bible.

Contents

Preface

In the beginning God created the heavens and the earth and all living things. He then gave to mankind a simple diet, one that was specifically designed for us. He then showed the human race the way to live and the path of salvation through Jesus Christ. Jesus' teachings and example lead to a simple, natural life.

This book explains why the first diet ever given to mankind is the best possible diet for us. It describes the many health dangers of our current ways of eating and why they must be changed. It describes how diseases come about and how they are healed by foods that have the powers to heal, foods that are tailored to our biological makeup. It explores the supernatural design and spiritual significance of this diet. It provides the incentives and encouragement needed to change not only our diets, but the very way that we live. So strong are the effects that foods have on our lives.

The evidence against the foods that are most commonly eaten in this country and throughout the world is so overwhelming that it is surprising that anyone would continue to eat them, especially when there are so many other foods that have been proven to promote and sustain optimum health and reduce the chances of getting diseases and other health issues.

We need look no further for proof of the destructiveness of most of the diets of the world than the rising incidence of heart disease, cancer, kidney disease, diabetes and a host of other life-shortening sicknesses, some of which were unknown only a few decades ago. The same is true for joint-related diseases, such as arthritis, bursitis, ankylosing spondylitis, avascular necrosis and gout. All are increasing in this country and in the world.

A Christian Diet

Imagine a vine branch deciding to live apart from the vine. Could the branch ever grow leaf or fruit? Of course not. Yet, we are likewise interfering with the best use of the life we have by eating foods that are detrimental to health.

Despite the billions of dollars of federal, state and private money spent each year searching for cures for human diseases, the diseases continue to prevail. But this does not make us change our diets. Many of us still eat the same foods we have always eaten. But many dietary studies and clinical trials conducted on human health closely link health disorders of every kind with faulty dietary practices, practices that cause internal poisoning of the organs and tissues of the body, poisoning that manifests itself in the outward signs (symptoms) of diseases.

I began my journey to optimum health by reading about foods and nutrition after years of consuming harmful foods and drinks and seeing the effects that they had on my health and the health of others. By explaining the effect of diet change on health, and by attempting to answer some of the most crucial questions relating to health, I hope to bring readers through a process of exploration and understanding that I myself went through.

This book explores many long-held beliefs about health that many of us take for granted, such as allowing cultural norms and traditions to dictate what foods we should eat, and seeing a doctor whenever we are sick. It describes the many health dangers of our current ways of eating and why they must be changed. It provides information of vital importance for the attainment of health in this most crucial century. Our neglect of the foods that God intended for us to eat has brought about the woeful health conditions that are so prevalent in the world today.

Anyone who has a health disorder, such as a disease, has it for a reason. When the cause and effect relationship between a health disorder and what we are doing to ourselves becomes apparent to us, then the best solution will be known, as well as the proper steps that are needed to put it into effect.

Ordinary diets, chaotic and haphazard food combining and unhealthy food cravings produce sickness. But a diet of life-giving foods, and the other practices that are described in this book enable the body to heal itself of practically any health disorder, including cancer, heart disease and the many lesser ailments of which humankind is susceptible.

The book is for anyone who is interested in improving their health. It is for the seeker of truth about foods and nutrition. It is for those who have many years ahead of them who want to remain healthy and enjoy the best out of life. It is for those who perhaps have no other choice than to begin learning about foods and nutrition at a late age, who realize that if they do not do something about their health then only worse days are ahead for them.

God knows what is best for us. When we abide in His Word, we allow ourselves to live as He intended for us to live.

Introduction

We are now experiencing a heightened awareness in this country and in the world of the many health hazards that are associated with eating certain foods. The traditional, or standard American, diet is the most commonly practiced diet in the Western world. It consists of high intakes of cooked foods, including meats, dairy products, eggs, refined grain products, jarred, canned and bottled fruits and vegetables, fractionated oils, refined sugar and refined salt. This diet is known to cause many of the diseases and health issues that are prevalent in the world today.

It is with great humility that I write this book. An engineer by training, I am more used to dealing with facts and figures than anything else. The Holy Scriptures and the important subject of human health have been my guiding lights for many years. It is from the study of both that this book is written.

I began reading the Bible after suffering a career setback that pulled the rug out from under me at age 42. I had always been interested in foods and nutrition, for my mother was a nutritionist, but it struck me how significantly God's decree for us in His Word agrees with what nutritionists and nutrition-minded medical doctors have been telling us for years about what foods we should eat for health and longevity.

As a Christian, I am concerned about what I should do for God that would please Him. But besides our honored duty to love and obey Him and try to live out our lives as ambassadors of Christ, what other things does He expect us to do?

It must be remembered that God seeks expression in the human race, for He works in us to will and to do for His good pleasure.

He works in us and through us to accomplish His will. It would seem, therefore, that health issues that adversely affect us in the ways that they do, such as weakening the immune system, destroying our capacity to be effective in the world and distracting us from what we are trying to do, should be adequately dealt with.

Joshua's wars were won by God. But Israel had to fight them. God helps us in the battles of life, but we must do our part. As portrayed in the gospel story about the loaves and fishes, He blesses our actions, but only after we make the required efforts.

To ensure that our work, God's work through us, is best carried out, we should keep watch not only over our souls but our health. When we are as healthy as we can be, the work or endeavor that God has given to us will not be weakened or hindered in anyway by health issues. It is then that we can be the most useful to our fellowman.

However, many Christians do not consider their health to be a top priority. By putting other things first, many end up compromising on their health. It is compounded by a common misconception that can lead to a resignation about health issues. It is not unusual for Christians to think that their health problems are brought on by God, either for sins committed (John 9:1), testing of faith (James 1:2-3; 1 Pet. 1:7) or chastening (Heb. 12:7-12). As a result, some of us are more inclined to acquiesce to health issues than take the proper steps that would remedy or cure them.

God indeed tests our faith and chastens those whom He loves. But chastening can take on many forms, and perhaps each is chosen to have a unique effect on the individual's growth and well-being. With the exception of being cast down and stricken by God for purposes of bringing us to our knees and to repentance, it is hard for me to believe that a holy God desires that man, His favorite creation, should suffer illness, disease and premature death when His rod and His staff comforts us (Ps. 23), and each of us already suffers, and will continue to suffer, in many ways because of our inadequacies and sins.

I believe that we must never let unanswered prayer come between us and the goodness of God.

It has been my experience and observation that we are more than capable of causing our own sicknesses. We unwittingly bring sickness and disease upon ourselves through dietary practices that are contrary to the laws of nature. The body requires a variety of nutrients to keep itself in health, but seldom finds them in the foods that are commonly eaten. It requires enzymes for proper digestion, but they are destroyed by heat, and almost all refined and processed foods are heat treated. Deprived of the nutrients and other essentials it needs to enhance the body's self-cleansing process, the natural law of cause and effect determines the outcome, which is ill-health.

He has given us a sound mind to figure things out (2 Tim. 1:7). Instead of believing that health problems are given to us as a penance or for atonement for past sins, we should learn all we can about how health problems arise, and then take the proper steps to rid ourselves of them. Although not in the Bible, an appropriate saying is, "God helps those who help themselves."

It is our responsibility to take care of our bodies. It is not our doctor's, our spouse's, our friends' or the Government's. It is our responsibility.

God put us here for a reason, to live to the utmost of our abilities, no matter what the difficulties or obstacles, by using what we were given at birth together with the skills that we acquire in life, and the tempered judgment that He bestows on us.

Perhaps we should pray not so much for the removal of a health issue as for the wisdom to know how to do something about it. Very often, all that is needed to resolve a health issue is to change something about the way that we are living. A change in diet is often required to correct a health issue. But with all the new fad diets coming out each year, and each one claiming to be the best yet for health, how are we to decide what is best for us?

The answer is simple, look to the Bible. Although the Bible may not explain all that we may wish that it did, or answer everything that we may want answers for, it provides us with many ineffable precepts and truths that have served as foundations for the establishment of universal human rights, our democratic government, the laws of the land and the criminal justice system. It has been the impetus for the abolitionists' argument for the dissolution of slavery, the women's suffrage argument for equal pay and voting rights, the argument against child labor and the argument against abortion.

The Bible tells us what we need to know in order to live properly in the world, and that includes diet. It also tells us many things about the saints of old and about Jesus and the apostles who fasted and ate sparingly. It shows us how Jesus' example and teachings lead to a simpler life, one that is better for us in numerous ways.

While written through human agency, the Bible is known to be the inspired Word of God, containing what God wants His favorite creation to know.

How Eating Habits Are Formed

Let's start with the basics. I have often found it beneficial to examine the things that are taken for granted, especially when it comes to foods and nutrition.

Whether young or old, male or female, the main criterion for food choices for most people is how foods taste and go down rather than how they affect health. In other words, taste-appeal over health-appeal. Unfortunately, this truth has been exploited by the many concerns of the food industry in the creation of many substances that are added to our foods and drinks to make them more appetizing.

The second basis for food selection is the emotional pulls that certain foods have on us. Both of these food selection reasons drive the majority of our decisions about foods. They also cause food habits to form.

Food habits are long-standing patterns of behavior associated with eating. Those of us who grew up on burgers, French fries and soft drinks tend to stick with that menu, or slight variations of it, throughout life, unless of course change is initiated.

It is now evident to most people that many of the health disorders prevalent in this country and throughout the world are diet-related. However, many of us continue to eat just as we did last year and the year before because of our habits. Another reason is that we have been culturally indoctrinated to believe that certain foods, such as meat and dairy products, sugary foods and drinks, and refined and processed foods, are good for us. Both pressures are reducing our numbers rapidly. Eating foods that we grew up on is not working.

A Christian Diet

A habit once formed and persistently practiced eventually turns into a craving, whether for chocolates, ice cream, sweet rolls or anything else. The worst part of cravings is that they stay with us even when they are doing us harm. Food cravings are encouraged by the many advertisements in the media for foods and drinks. Despite their oftentimes silky persuasiveness, the products being sold are, for the most part, refined and processed foods and drinks that have been heat treated, chemically altered, devitalized and robbed of precious nutrients. Not surprisingly, many of the ads support the meat, dairy and grain interests, the chief vested interests in our food industry.

But anyone with a little persistence and willpower can change their eating habits, or for that matter any other habit in life. Voluntary change begins in the mind. Healthy eating habits are formed when we become convinced that dietary change is in our best interests.

However, many people believe that they are, and have been, living healthy lives, and in particular, they believe that they are eating healthy foods, even when they have health issues. But this is belied when the causes of disease and lesser health disorders are examined, as we will see in a subsequent chapter.

I grew up at the time when fast-food franchises were just starting out in this country. I was hooked on, and for years ate the foods of the Standard American Diet. But as I learned more and more about foods and nutrition, and saw the ill effects that the diet had on myself and others, I began eating healthier foods.

People in this country should be the healthiest people on earth. It certainly seems that way since there are now more varieties of health-promoting and sustaining foods available to us than ever before, and many of them are organically grown. But we are not the healthiest people because of our preferences for artificial, man-made foods and drinks, our giving way to cultural norms and traditions about foods, and our unwillingness, even refusal, to abide by Nature's laws that govern health and well-being.

By choosing to ignore the information that has been gained in the human health field which proves that diseases and a host of lesser human ailments are caused by commonly eaten foods, many of us are sacrificing our health for eating habits and food cravings. But the remarkable truth is that eating habits can be changed, even when food cravings exist, and that everyone is capable of changing their diet in enlightened self-interest.

The Body

The body is a marvelously powerful healing organism capable of healing itself of diseases, restoring to health any ill-health condition and releasing its rejuvenating powers into action, but only if it is properly cared for, as we shall see in this book.

When supplied with the life-supporting nourishment and other pro-health things that it needs, the body can remain in optimum health for much longer than the average human lifespan. It is designed for stupendous feats and deeds, as we observe throughout the world. The body's amazing resilience and its many capabilities far out-marvel anything made by humankind. Yet in many ways it is fragile and utterly dependent on its caretaker for its needs.

The healing powers of the body are fully at work when we live in concert with the laws of Nature. But when we depart from Nature's laws by putting foods in us that harm the body, or do other things that are bad for health such as depriving the body of adequate exercise, sunshine, fresh air and rest. we court disaster in the form of disease or some other troublesome health issue. However, if we understand the laws of Nature and abide by them, illness and disease are vanquished by the body's inherent life-promoting and life-sustaining powers.

Nutritional experts and nutrition-minded doctors stress that sickness and disease cannot exist in a body that has cleansed itself of acidic and toxic wastes by the powers of living, whole plant foods, the foods that are most conducive to human health, the foods that have the powers to heal. These foods allow us to trade our sorrows and disappointments for joy and gladness, and enable us to live simpler and more enjoyable lives. Adopting a whole plant food diet and restricting food intake to manageable amounts of the most easily digestible foods helps to ensure that every seed of sickness is extirpated from the body.

The Causes of Disease

"To the degree that foods are used in their completely natural state, without treatment or processing, are they adapted to support life and maintain immunity to disease." - Arnold Paul De Vries.

Diseases seem to wait in ambush, ready to strike and slay. But what are they really, at least according to our best scientific understanding, and what does this understanding tell us about how diseases may be cured? This chapter explores these topics.

There are, no doubt, hundreds of diseases that afflict humankind, including all the fevers, tumors and contagion of human life   It is not the purpose of this book to chronicle all human diseases or to give an account of the known causes of them, but to explore some of the attempts made by man to understand, control and cure the diseases that beset him. Two views of diseases will be presented, the view commonly held by the mainstream medical profession, and the view held by modern nutritionists.

Bear in mind that since human diseases appear to have certain causes, and there are methods by which they can be avoided, there must be ways to cure them.

Mainstream Medicine View

The deadliest diseases in this country, and the most feared, are heart disease; cancer of the organs, including colon, bladder, lung and breast cancer, kidney disease, and the neurological diseases, including Alzheimer's disease and Parkinson's disease. According to mainstream medicine, the causes of these diseases are primarily foreign substances, including but not limited to bacteria, viruses and poisons that get into, or invade, the body. The theory of infection is built around micro-organisms; in short, micro-biology, a product of laboratory work based on the proposition that micro-organisms, which include bacteria and viruses, are responsible for the majority of our diseases. The attempts made by mainstream medicine to cure diseases are primarily efforts that are aimed at eradicating the foreign substances and organisms that are believed to cause the diseases.

The methods used by mainstream medicine to treat diseases include pharmaceutical drugs, antibiotics such as penicillin and erythromycin, and medical intervention such as hospitalization and surgery. Many of the drugs must be improved yearly by medical laboratories to counteract the proliferation of drug-resistant organisms that result from their use. Chemotherapy and radiation therapy are used. Vaccines may also be used. These methods are, for the most part, all that mainstream medicine has in its arsenal against diseases.

Standard medical treatments focus on achieving health through drugs. For headaches, take aspirin or a similar product; for stomachaches or heartburn, take antacids; for infections, take antibiotics; for constipation, take laxatives; for cancer, take chemotherapy or radiation therapy. But even considering drugs like penicillin which can halt the spread of a disease, drugs do not possess the ability to cure, and there are risks associated with all drugs. Also, drugs have been known to lodge in the system for decades after their use[1].

Diseases which are today considered eradicated, such as malaria, smallpox and poliomyelitis, are not eradicated in the true sense of

---

[1] From the book, <u>Prof. Arnold Ehret's Mucusless Diet Healing System: Annotated, Revised, and Edited by Prof. Spira</u>.

the word, because the viruses or parasites associated with them still exist. They are merely prevented from causing excessive harm through vaccination, which is the most common form of immunization used against diseases.

There are, of course, exceptions. Leprosy and inflammation of the eyes (uveitis, a disease that can cause blindness), can both be cured through drug therapy, unless, in the case of eye inflammation, the cause is an autoimmune disorder. Both diseases were the scourge of the Middle East 200 years ago when many of the population suffered terribly from them. Physical blindness today is often prevented merely through sanitary measures.

Permanent cures of diseases by mainstream medicine are rare.[2] It is believed that many of the cures that are attributed to mainstream medical treatments would have occurred naturally without them.

Furthermore, as evidenced in hospitals throughout the world, many patients of chronic and acute diseases die despite the treatments they receive, or even because of them. In 2014, in the United States and Europe, prescription drugs were the third leading cause of death, after heart disease and cancer. In 2016, a John Hopkins University study indicated that the third leading cause of death in this country was medical errors.

---

[2] For example, the average cure rate for all types of cancer by mainstream medicine, except for skin cancer, is 17% per G. Edmond Griffin's book, World Without Cancer. It is believed to be more like 6% per Rich Anderson's book, Cleanse & Purify Thyself. A 2019 American Cancer Society Web article states that most cancers cannot be cured, but some can be controlled for months or even years. A cancer.net article sponsored by the American Society of Clinical Oncology (ASCO) states that chronic cancer is cancer that cannot be cured.

These things have led many people to seek second or even third opinions about their health issues. Blind faith in the medical profession has eroded since the earlier days, but many are not finding suitable alternatives, nor have they gained sufficient knowledge about foods and nutrition to convince themselves that dietary change is necessary and the need to take charge of their own health is paramount.

Mainstream medicine spends billions of dollars of federal, state and private funds each year trying to find cures for diseases, especially the top 10 deadliest diseases in this country. But cures for these diseases remain elusive. Despite continuing assurances from medical research labs that cures are in the offing (which, by the way, has been going on for quite some time), it is doubtful whether cures will be realized as long as the underlying causes of disease are believed to be foreign substances or organisms.

To effectively deal with any disease, the underlying cause, or causes, of the disease must be known. Mainstream medicine's attempts at curing diseases have not met with success in the vast majority of cases, including the top t0 leading causes of death in this country, which strongly suggests that the causes that are commonly attributed to diseases are not really the underlying causes at all, but only contributing causes or factors that can localize a disease to certain parts of the body.

It appears that disease will remain, at least for the present, somewhat of a mystery to mainstream medicine, maybe as much of a mystery as disease was to the "medicine man" of yesteryear. Having directed its energies and skills primarily at the suppression of the symptoms of diseases, mainstream medicine appears to have missed the mark, as we shall see.

The Nutritionist View

Nutritional experts do not believe that "germs" or bacteria and viruses are the primary causes of disease. Rather, it is the presence of undigested and uneliminated rotting food waste accumulated over time in the tissues and organs of the body due to eating wrong kinds of foods and overeating. In their view, these things mean that elimination of the foul material is the only rational means of curing disease.

"In food lies 99.99% of the causes of all disease and imperfect health of any kind. Consequently, all healing, all therapeutics will continue to fail as long as they refuse to place the most important stress on diet." - Arnold Ehret, *Mucusless Diet Healing System*.

Viruses and bacteria are everywhere and exist in everyone, but before they can proliferate and thrive in the body, they must have suitable soil. Nutritionists believe that it is the waste material in the body that affords the germs the suitable soil for them to proliferate and produce the symptoms of disease.

Many nutritionists, including those who are referenced in this book, contend that almost all human diseases are the result of internal poisoning, typically organ or blood poisoning, that occurs when the tissues of the body become congested with toxic waste material due to constipation. They believe that disease symptoms are manifested as a result of this poisoning, and that they are signs the body gives when it attempts to eliminate the poisons. Malaise and fatigue are two typical signs of internal poisoning.

In other words, disease is an attempt to rid the organism of the foul material with which it is contaminated. Also, disease symptoms are the outward manifestation of an automatic internal bodily cleansing process. For example, nausea and fever result from the body's natural attempts to rid itself of morbid, toxic material that has accumulated in the tissues. They are not due to "infectious organisms" that invade the body.

The cure for disease, then, is not to treat the symptoms, including the pains that may result from the disease, but the underlying causes of the symptoms. Nutritionists contend that it is the only way the body can rid itself of disease, recover and resume a life of health. If the natural self-healing process is repressed through medication (drugs), and we continue the consumption of foods and drinks that are harmful to the body, then the cure is thwarted.

"The foods you consume can heal you faster and more profoundly than the most expensive prescription drugs, and more dramatically than the most extreme surgical interventions, with only positive side effects. They can prevent cancer, heart disease, Type 2 diabetes, stroke, macular degeneration, migraines, erectile dysfunction, and arthritis – and that's only the short list." - T. Colin Campbell and Howard Jacobson, *Whole, Rethinking the Science of Nutrition.*

Furthermore, mainstream medicine places emphasis on treating specific, localized symptoms. Modern drugs are prescribed to correct one symptom or another without effectively strengthening the overall state of health. But the body is an integral organism consisting of many parts, with every part connected with every other part. All parts of the body receive the same blood and lymphatic fluid supply to support its needs. No one part can be diseased and the rest be healthy. Similarly, when one or more parts of the body are healed of ill-health, the other parts of the body benefit as well.

According to nutritional experts, local treatments are harmful to the entire body, not just the part or parts that may be displaying the symptoms. They contend that almost all attempts made by mainstream medicine to cure diseases are not successful in a true sense, but can, at best, only forestall the diseases from taking over and killing the patients in the short term.

Medications can temporarily relieve pains and inhibit inflammation, but they can weaken the immune system, and are often habit forming. Many of the published medical books and articles available to us about human diseases reveal that patients must often cope with the toxicity of the substances that are prescribed for their illness as well as the illness itself.

As powerful as the medical profession is, it seems to have eyes that cannot see and ears that cannot hear in its quest for cures for diseases. Because of this, we are in danger of being continually affected in adverse ways by medical treatments as time goes by.

As emphasized throughout this book, when confronted with a health issue, we should do everything in our power to resolve it without resorting to doctors. When the cause and effect relationship between a health issue and what we are doing to ourselves becomes apparent to us, the best solution will then be known, as well as the proper steps that are needed to put it into effect.

Healing does not come from drugs. It comes from natural bodily processes, such as self-cleansing or detoxification that remove accumulated toxins, obstructions and acidosis from the body, from rest, and from providing the body with the nourishment it needs.

The beacon of warning, the clarion call for proper action, has been sent out. We need to become more our own doctors than ever before, and the sooner it starts the better it will be for us, to avoid the unnecessary suffering associated with medical treatments that are not designed to heal.

I suffered from various physical ailments for years that caused me a lot of pain and suffering. However, in each case, I tried my best to search out the answers to what caused them, and the knowledge I gained allowed me to determine how to cure them. When the conditions were sufficiently understood, I took what I believed were the proper steps to resolve them.

One may wonder, as I did, why we do not all get diseases, such as polio, diphtheria, typhoid or cholera. The answer from a nutritionist's viewpoint is that there is no suitable soil in our bodies in which these diseases can take root. It appears to be the only reason we do not all get diseases. Micro-organisms cannot harm us as long as our organism functions in a normal, healthy way. Microbes and viruses are harmless if the body's defensive mechanisms, including the immune system, are in good working order.

What if a person already has a disease? How then may he or she be cured? According to nutritional experts, if a person already has a disease but deprives the micro-organisms their food and renders the human soil unsuitable for their growth, then the disease can be cured. From this perspective, there is hope that disease may not only be prevented, but cured through natural means.

Disease should not be looked on as an affliction brought on by fate or Providence, but something primarily, or perhaps even solely, brought on by an ignorance of the unalterable laws of nature, and most notably the laws governing foods and nutrition.[3]

The body's ability to fight illnesses is determined by the health of the immune system. Certain diseases, including cancer, repress the immune system and allow increased attacks by unfriendly microbes and viruses. Nutritionists tell us that the best way to improve the health of the immune system is to eat whole plant foods.

"A whole food plant-based diet deals with so many diseases and conditions that you begin to wonder if there isn't just one basic disease cause – poor nutrition – that manifests through thousands of different symptoms...Poor nutrition causes vastly more diseases than the disease care system currently acknowledges; but good nutrition, in contrast, is a cure for all those diseases and more." - T. Colin Campbell and Howard Jacobson, *Whole, Rethinking the Science of Nutrition*.

Bear in mind, however, that no cure can be expected to work while eating habits are constantly counteracting the cure.

Mucus-forming Foods

Professor Arnold Ehret, a nutritionist popular in Germany in the early 1900s and later in America, was probably the first to recognize that mucus-forming foods cause waste obstruction in the body, and that the obstruction causes disease. In his book,

---

[3] If fasting can cure almost all diseases of which the human race is susceptible, and it can as we shall see in the chapter on "The Importance of Fasting," then what does it tell us about how diseases and other health disorders originate? Doesn't it clearly reveal that the principle cause of almost all human maladies lies in the foods that are eaten? Does it not assuredly implicate improper diet as the main cause of our many ailments?

A Christian Diet

The Cause and Cure of Human Illness, he states that there are two main reasons for human disease: 1) constipation caused by mucus-producing foods, and 2) overeating, i.e., eating more than is necessary, more than the system actually needs -- more calories than the body needs.

Mucusless foods are non-starchy foods. They include raw fruits, leafy greens and non-starchy vegetables.

Ehret healed himself of Bright's disease (a kidney disease), and cured many hopeless cases of chronic diseases by putting his patients on his mucusless diet and fasting regimen. Many of the patients were very serious cases with terminal diseases, and lay on their deathbeds. Many had gone through other therapies, including those requiring strict diets, but without success. He also cured those who suffered from degenerative diseases, both acute and chronic. After following his mucusless diet for only a short time, all of his patients regained their health. Can conventional medicine, with its use of pharmaceutical drugs and/or medical intervention, including surgery and chemotherapy that are intended to cure diseases, make such claims?

Ehret believed that the buildup of mucus in the body was the first and foremost cause of disease, and that health can only be restored when the buildup is removed from the body. He did not claim that mucus was the only cause of every disease, but that it was the main cause present in almost all diseases.

"There is no man in existence in western civilization whose body has not been continually stuffed since childhood with cow milk, meat and eggs, potatoes and cereal products." - Arnold Ehret, *Mucusless Diet Healing System*.

In his landmark book, *The Mucusless Diet Healing System*, first published in 1922, Ehret released to the world his incredible findings regarding a starch-free diet consisting of raw fresh fruits, leafy greens and non-starchy vegetables (mucusless foods) which he claimed was the optimal diet for human health. The book is considered by many nutritionists to be the definitive work on the prevention and curing of human disease through diet and fasting.

Ehret's book has become one of the most important texts in the modern raw food movement. Raw food eaters have repeatedly confirmed that the mucusless diet heals diseases.

As revealed in many of the books that are listed in the Bibliography, it is the firm conviction of many nutritionists that starchy foods, which are mucus-producing foods, cause human disease. The reason for this is explained in the chapter on "The Dangers of Starchy Foods."

The body attempts to rid itself of mucus through the lymphatic system which typically results in various forms of expulsion or expectoration, such as excessive saliva, clearing of the throat, coughing, sneezing, colds, flus, and congestion of the lungs, throat and ears. Nutritionists believe that these are all signs of excessive mucus in the body.

"All disease is finally, nothing else but a clogging up of the smallest blood vessels, the capillaries, by mucus." - Arnold Ehret, *Rational Fasting and Roads to Health and Happiness.*

Berg's Tables, which appear in Appendix I, list what foods are acid-binding and acid-forming. These terms are synonymous with mucus-binding and mucus-forming, respectively. The most mucus-producing foods are meat and grain products, whereas fruits and vegetables are the most mucus-binding foods.

When the large intestine, or colon, becomes obstructed, it hinders the absorption of nutrients in the body. Poor nutrient absorption leads to nutrient deficiency. If the food is nutrient-deficient in the first place, then even less nutrients are assimilated by the body.

If true, then we live in a very sick world, a world in which almost everyone is addicted to mucus-producing cooked and starchy foods, with their devitalizing properties and adverse effects on heath.

Again, Professor Ehret:

"Disease is an effort of the body to eliminate waste, mucus and toxemias, and the system assists nature in the most perfect and natural way. Not the disease but the body is to be healed, it must be cleansed, freed from waste and foreign matter, from mucus and toxemias accumulated since childhood. You cannot buy health in a bottle, you cannot heal your body, that is, cleanse your system, in a few days, you must make "compensation" for the wrong you have done your body all during your life." - Arnold Ehret, *Mucusless Diet Healing System*.

According to nutritionist Robert Morse, mucus-forming foods are responsible for many types of inflammation in the body, such as the diseases that end in "itis", including bursitis and arthritis.

Obesity

We have an obesity epidemic in this country. It is due to several factors, not all of which will be discussed in this book, but the main factors will be covered. One of the main causes for the epidemic is the consumption of saturated fats found in cooked foods, including, but not limited to, meat and dairy products and refined and processed snack foods. Because cooked foods are deficient in nutrients and enzymes, our hunger is not satisfied when we eat cooked foods, so we overeat, which compounds the problem.

It is well known that the more obese a person is, the more likely he or she will become a victim of disease. Overeating is so common in the US that it's considered "normal," even though it is a precursor of many health complications.

Overeating contributes to the wastes that build up in the body. Nutritionists, such as Dr. Robert Morse, believe that digestive juices are secreted not in proportion to the amount of food eaten, but in proportion to the amount of food that is required by the system. This may change your opinion about overeating.

As an obese person, or any other person, continues to overeat, their system becomes more and more clogged up, choked with internal undigested waste material. The resulting putrefaction causes bodily acidity and produces toxins that pollute the blood (bodily toxicity).

Gluttony can cause obesity. The dictionary defines gluttony as habitual greed or excess in eating. Instead of overeating because the body senses a lack of nutrients in the foods, the glutton desires more food just for the sake of it.

From a science of nutrition point of view, gluttony may be defined as habitually eating in excess of the body's supply of gastric juices. The Bible frowns on gluttony, treating it like drunkenness.

Overeating is so widespread that I sought additional reasons that might explain the epidemic. One of the reasons appears to be the pride or hubris that is associated with having a plentiful supply of foods. We don't face starvation in this country, just the choice between a Whopper and a Big Mac. We have more food than anyone needs or can possibly use, and in such an unrivaled variety of products. It is a supply that others in the world do not have. So, why pass up the opportunity to indulge, while you still can? Such thinking leads us into ill-health.

A Slightly Different View of Diseases

Some nutritionists believe that diseases are best explained as the result of three causes. The first two are brought about by the practice of consuming foods and drinks that are harmful to the body, or the practice of combining foods improperly. The third is what some consider to be a possible cause of diseases.

1. Toxicity

2. Acidity

3. Heredity / Genes

Let's examine each.

Toxicity

Toxicity is internal poisoning that is brought about by accumulated waste material in the body. According to nutritionists, it is the most common ill-health condition prevalent today. It is mainly the result of eating the wrong foods, such as animal-based foods that are baked or deep-fried in oils; starchy foods, including doughnuts, sweet rolls, pasta and bread; and other refined and processed, heat-treated foods, including canned, jarred and most packaged snack foods. Toxicity results from the morbid accumulation of toxins and food wastes in the organs and tissues of the body, and is similar to mucus buildup from eating mucus-producing foods.

Secondary causes of toxicity of the body include the ingestion of chemical preservatives and man-made additives that are found in refined and processed foods, and the ingestion of pesticide residues on foods. Common medical practices also cause toxicity of the body, such as vaccinations and prescription drugs.

Poisons can also get into the body from the environment, from municipal drinking water, car exhaust fumes, cigarette smoke, and toxic chemicals that we become exposed to in the home and on the job. All contribute to the toxicity of the body. Some of these pollutants are carcinogenic or mutagenic. It seems very likely that exposure to these toxic substances will continue for some time to come in our society.

The result is that the body is made toxic by substances it ingests or is exposed to. The good news is that certain foods, such as green leafy vegetables, protect us from the harmful effects of carcinogens like no drug can. Chlorophyll in green plants detoxifies the liver and bloodstream and neutralizes environmental pollutants. To receive this protection, all we need to do is include greens in our diet.

Many people take inorganic substances in the form of multivitamin/mineral supplements on a daily basis. Billions of dollars are spent each year in America alone on these substances. Also, many take medication every day as prescribed by their doctors. Inorganic substances and drugs are not properly utilized by the body but are treated by the body as toxins. Many of them get stored in the body's tissues.

Some of the internal damage caused by toxic substances heals automatically. But when overloaded with toxins, the body cannot eliminate the poisons fast enough, which causes them to accumulate in the tissues. And that is when they can cause harm, such as weakening the immune system.

Commonly consumed foods, including meat, fish, eggs, and dairy products, contain substances that are toxic or otherwise harmful to the body, including carcinogens, hormones, dioxins, bacteria, and other contaminants that can accumulate in your body and remain there for years. Every year we hear of meat products contaminated with E. coli, listeria, campylobacter, or other dangerous bacteria that live in the intestinal tracts, flesh, and feces of animals.

Other commonly consumed food products contain substances that are known to be harmful to human health, including table salt, refined sugar, hydrogenated oils, preservatives, artificial colors and sweeteners, excitotoxins such as monosodium glutamate (MSG) and GMO (Genetically Modified Organism) food products such as High Fructose Corn Syrup (HFCS). All are unnatural substances produced by man-made processes.

Evidence from X-rays and autopsies of people with long histories of poor eating habits, such as eating a lot of cooked and starchy foods, reveals a plaster-like coating formed on the inner surfaces of the large intestine, or colon. This coating, or what many investigators call "plaque", prevents foods from being fully digested and assimilated, and often causes obstruction of the colon. In time, the coating builds up to where the intestines become mostly or even totally obstructed. A thorough discussion of intestinal obstruction, with sketches, is found in Dr. Norman W. Walker's book, *Become Younger.*

The colon is the septic tank of the body. It needs to be cleaned out periodically for health. But if this is not attended to, and foods which are harmful to the body continue to be eaten, toxification of the entire organism is the result causing not only cancers but many types of serious health disorders such as stroke. The consensus of many modern nutritionists, including those whose books are listed in the Bibliography, is that internal poisoning and morbidity are precursors of illness and disease.

Self-cleansing or detoxification is what removes accumulated toxins from the body. More about detoxification in a subsequent chapter.

Constipation is a major cause of internal toxicity. It is worsened by the rapid growth of parasites that thrive and flourish in the rotting intestinal wastes. Stopped up wastes are a fertile breeding ground for many kinds of non-friendly parasites, including tapeworms which can cause many complications. A person may have a bowel movement once a day and think that everything is fine, but everything is not fine.

One bowel movement a day is a sign of a serious health concern. It is a warning signal given by the body that something is wrong and should be corrected as soon as possible. Foods that are devoid of fiber, such as meats, dairy and white flour products, are known to cause constipation.

When in good health, one can expect to have as many bowel movements per day as meals taken per day. It is one of the gauges used for telling whether a person is in good health. Real freedom, no matter where you may be living, is constipated-free eliminations, probably the best comfort you can ever have.

Toxic wastes continue to build up until corrective action is taken. To avoid suffering from toxic waste health disorders, the most important thing we can do is to reduce or eliminate the intake of foods and supplements that cause the toxic waste buildup, and eat raw plant foods instead. Antioxidant-rich foods are known to stop or even reverse toxic buildup. Whole plant foods are high in antioxidants that neutralize the poisons and help to flush them out of the system.

"A pure raw plant diet assists the body's cleansing efforts in the most natural way by eliminating any toxicity from entering the system and by simultaneously moving toxicity through the lymph and blood and out the body through the eliminating organs (the bowels, kidneys, liver, skin, sinuses and lungs). A purification of the diet enforces a self-healing and radical whole-body rejuvenation." - David Wolfe, *The Sunfood Diet Success System*.

Acidity

Acidity is a blood condition mainly brought on by eating acid-forming foods, such as cooked foods, but alcohol, caffeine and drugs (medication) also create acidity in the body. According to leading nutritionists, acid-forming foods are responsible for many of the diseases and health issues and that are prevalent in the world today, including diabetes and kidney failure.

Refined grain and cereal products, refined sugar, meat products, including sausages and hot dogs of beef or pork, and pasteurized dairy products are widely eaten today. All leave behind a residue of toxic acids In the body. Modern refining techniques, including the use of high-temperature heat treatment and over-cooking, destroy the alkaline mineral salts found in natural foods that act to neutralize these acids.

If the acids go unchecked, they form hard acid deposits in the system. The soft tissues of the body, including those in the throat and anus, are the first affected. Eventually, the acids are deposited in the muscles, joints and ligaments of the body, which can cause arthritis and many other diseases such as bursitis, colitis and diverticulitis.

Cooked foods create acidity in the body, whereas uncooked (raw) plant foods alkalize the body. Acidity in the body also occurs when foods are combined incorrectly. Foods improperly combined inhibit digestion and cause discomforts such as stomachache, abdominal pain and fermentation and gas. More about this in the chapter on "Proper Food Combinations."

Acid-forming foods include foods high in protein, such as eggs and beans as well as meat and dairy products. High protein foods cause the nutrients to stick together, which leads to cellular starvation and death. The foods also cause mucus production in the body, which is considered a forerunner of disease.

"People are becoming more and more acid. The public is not told this because the powers that be do not want people to know what is being done to them. In the last few decades, this fatal condition appears to be on the increase." - Rich Anderson, *Cleanse & Purify Thyself.*

Homeostasis is the tendency of the body to maintain itself in stable chemical equilibrium. It is the process whereby the body tries to balance or stabilize itself from an acidic condition to a normal alkaline condition.[4] Obviously, the effectiveness of the body's ability at doing this is encumbered or enhanced by the foods that are eaten.

---

[4] Robert Morse, N.D., The Detox Miracle Sourcebook.

An acidic blood condition often results from a nutrient deficient diet, such as the standard American diet. If the diet is continued, the blood condition worsens to where the body's attempts at homeostasis are not sufficient in neutralizing the acids. Toxic acids the body cannot expel as waste in its on-going self-cleansing efforts are stored in the tissues and joints which can lead to diseases.

Vegetables, including leafy greens, carrots, cabbage, tomatoes, raw nuts, seeds and Superfoods, are alkalizing to the body, creating an alkaline blood condition that is conducive to healing and regeneration.

Of all the foods that there are for us to eat, most people eat refined and processed foods, such as fast foods, canned and jarred foods, packaged bread and grain products, such as cereals, sweet rolls and pastries, packaged meat products including steaks, sausages, bacon, ham, hot dogs and hamburgers, and dairy products including milk, cream and cheese products.

Refined and processed foods have been heat treated (cooked) and almost always contain refined salt (table salt), refined and processed ingredients such as high fructose corn syrup (HFCS) and monosodium glutamate (MSG), and man-made flavors, colors and preservatives, none of which are natural products.

Americans eat more cooked food than any people on earth, and spend more money on doctor bills and healthcare than any people on earth. The fast food franchises, as well as other eating ootablishments, grill, fry, bake, steam-heat their foods, or use dehydrated foods that have already been refined and processed using these methods. It has been known for years that these methods destroy important food components such as enzymes, vitamins and other nutrients, and alter the chemical properties of the foods.

In contrast, nutritionists tell us that our bodies are biologically suited for alkaline-forming foods, which are the fruits and vegetables found in nature. Since these foods neutralize acids that can cause disease, heartburn, upset stomach, indigestion, flatulence and other complications, we need to eat plenty of these foods.

Acidic foods also contribute to, or can cause, diseases that end in "itis," including arthritis, bursitis, colitis and diverticulitis.

Stress produces acidity in the body. High levels of stress have been linked to all kinds of physical and mental disorders. This acid-producer seems to have taken up permanent residence in our society.

"You must remove the obstructions and acidosis, if you don't, the cause remains as you have treated only the effect which can be swelling, pain or other symptoms. These are nothing more than natural defenses of the body in response to the cause. De-toxification is the only logical answer that will yield a lasting cure. Alkalization is the method by which detoxification starts. Alkalization neutralizes acidosis. Detoxification not only alkalizes the body, but also gives the body the added energy it needs to clean itself." - Robert Morse, N.D., *The Detox Miracle Sourcebook*.

Berg's Tables, in Appendix I, list what foods are "acid-forming" and "acid-binding." According to these tables, meat and grain products are the most acid-forming foods, whereas fruits and vegetables are the most acid-binding foods.

Whenever we eat animal products, a particularly harmful acid is produced -- uric acid. Animal protein is complex protein that must be broken down before it can be assimilated by the body. The breaking down process results in the generation of an excessive amount of uric acid. Since the muscles of the body have an affinity for uric acid, it is initially deposited in the muscles. When the saturation point is reached and uric acid is sent to the kidneys, uric acid crystals are formed which can cause kidney stones and gout. According to Norman W. Walker's book, *Become Younger*, uric acid crystals can cause arthritis.

Nutritionists tell us that if we ate nothing but raw fruits and vegetables, our blood would be alkaline most of the time, except for periods of undue stress or when other causes of blood acidity are introduced.

The chapter on "The Blood" describes how blood tests are used in medical diagnosis in assessing the acidity of the body.

Heredity / Genes

Gregor Mendel, an Augustinian friar who lived in the 1800s in what is now the Czech Republic, is the founder of the science of genetics. He discovered dominant and recessive traits, and that parents can hand down a trait that is unlike themselves. He showed that a trait can be hidden for many generations and then become evident in offspring. Hence, scientists believe that people may have a proclivity for certain diseases because of their genetic makeup.

Scientists after Mendel have used his discoveries to help explain diseases that are believed to have a genetic basis. For example, it is believed that thin blood vessels of forefathers can have an effect on the lives of their offspring.

According to the National Human Genome Research Institute (NHGRI), an institute of the National Institutes of Health (NIH), genetic disorders are diseases caused by changes in the DNA due to mutations or damage to chromosomes.

Sickle cell anemia, a condition in which there are not enough healthy red blood cells to carry adequate oxygen throughout the body, is considered by the NHGRI to be an inherited disease. The reasons for this appear to be based on earlier work by scientists, such as Linus Pauling and Janet Watson on the molecular bases for sickle cell disease, which established the inheritance pattern of the disorder and of monogenic diseases in general, and later from a wide variety of experimental studies on mice involving DNA vectors and the development of gene delivery systems. The problem I see with this research is that it appears to assume rather than prove the conclusion that the disease is inherited. If you start off assuming a conclusion, you operate in a closed system.

The medical industry receives much of its funding for medical research from the NIH, which is part of the US Department of Health and Natural Resources. Many of the findings and positions of the Institute are based on the results of this research. It is speculative whether all the positions taken by the NIH, or for that matter the NHGRI, reflect views other than those of the medical industry. This is not to say that their findings should be dismissed, but that they should be viewed in a proper perspective.

Most scientists agree that certain physical characteristics, such as eye color and hair color, are inherited. But other characteristics, such as left-handedness, appear to have no biological basis.

Hand preference, for example, is believed to arise as part of the developmental process that differentiates the right and left sides of the body (called right-left asymmetry) which occurs at an early age.

Scientists have often speculated that certain disorders, such as mental aberrations or psychiatric disturbances, may have a biological or inherited basis. However, there appears to be no scientific proof or evidence of these things. It is now believed that environmental factors may contribute to such disturbances.

Some researchers say that genetic variations confer only a small risk of disease. The redoubtable Hereward Carrington in his book, *Vitality, Fasting and Nutrition*, observed that whenever disease, which he believed was the penalty of broken natural laws, is ascribed to heredity, we escape from taking responsibility for that disease. He preferred to ascribe diseases to being due to the simple fact that like causes produce like effects.

Heredity does not mean that we will get the diseases of our forefathers, even if we knew what they were, which most of us do not. It only means that we could get their diseases if, in fact, they were caused by genes, which is yet to be proven based on my researching.

The subject of inherited diseases is a controversial one. But despite the amount of detailed and extensive work that has been done by the medical profession on diseases, there has been very little, if any, scientific proof that any disease is caused by genetic deficiencies in DNA. Some diseases appear to have a biological basis, but the hard evidence is lacking to show they are the result of genes. There appears to be no consensus, either among modern medical researchers or nutritionists, that diseases that are ascribed to heredity are actually based on genetics. This may change in the future, but it appears to be the situation at the time of this writing.

"What you eat every day is a far more powerful determinant of your health than your DNA or most of the nasty chemicals lurking in your environment." - T. Colin Campbell and Howard Jacobson, *Whole, Rethinking the Science of Nutrition*.

Many of the diseases that afflict us appear to be the result of either an unwitting ignorance of the unalterable laws of nature, or a willful refusal to abide by these laws. Adopting a whole plant food diet and restricting food intake to manageable amounts of the most easily digestible foods helps to ensure that every seed of sickness is extirpated from the body.

"Man's health or his disease of every description, directly result from food intake. His state of mind may be a contributing factor, but the fall of mankind in the final analysis is "sin of diet." The real physiological cause of all evils, especially the physical ailments of mankind can be traced directly to the present day accepted diet of civilization." - Arnold Ehret, *Rational Fasting and Roads to Health and Happiness*.

As discussed in this chapter, disease, from a nutritionist point of view, is a consequence of something that is wrong with the organism. Contrary to the tenets of mainstream medicine, nutritionists believe that disease is a rational process of the body attempting to cure itself of excess acid or toxic waste that it should not have accumulated. The main cause of this accumulation is faulty diet which creates acidity or toxicity in the body and causes constipation which, in turn, causes unfriendly bacteria to proliferate inordinately in the waste material that results in blood poisoning by the toxins that are thereby produced. In either case, the primary cause is improper diet.

Improvements in health can be said to start when the vital roles of foods and nutrition in promoting human health are realized.

The God-given Diet

"And God said, "See, I have given you every herb that yields seed which is on the face of all the earth, and every tree whose fruit yields seed; to you it shall be for food." - Gen. 1:29.

In the beginning God created the heavens and the earth. He also gave to mankind a simple diet, one that was specifically designed for man. But after the Fall, the diet, like so many other oracles received from God, was soon abandoned as man chose to go his own way and do what was right in his own eyes.

The foods that man first ate were whole plant foods, the foods of Genesis 1:29. According to the Bible, man learned to eat foods that were inconsistent with his original diet only after his fall from grace. No mention of fire, or foods being cooked by fire, is made in the Scriptures during the time that man was in the Garden. It was after the Fall that man broke away from the diet given to him by God, and adopted other ways of eating. For example, it is only after the Fall that the Bible indicates that foods were prepared by fire.

The Fall changed our natures, but not the way the body was designed, nor did it change the body's nutritional requirements, the requirements that were perfectly met by whole plant foods.

A diet consisting of the foods of Genesis 1:29 is best described as the raw vegan diet. The raw vegan diet includes all raw fruits and vegetables, leafy greens (leafy green vegetables), nuts and seeds, grains and legumes. These foods may be eaten in any quantity desired. The diet excludes all animal-based foods (animal products), and all cooked foods.

Whole plant foods are different in many ways from other foods. Apples, when planted in the soil, produce additional apple trees. Raw nuts planted in the ground produce other nut trees. Even a harvested potato when planted yields at least another potato plant. But many of the foods that are consumed on ordinary diets have been devitalized by heat treatment. Cooking destroys the life force properties that are in whole plant foods. Plant a cooked bean or tomato or a roasted nut in the ground and it will not grow. Cooked foods, including refined and processed foods, do not promote or sustain health, but are harmful to the body.

The Creator has blessed and enriched the earth with a wide assortment of life-promoting plant foods. We live in a green world. Green is the color of nature, the symbol of youth and growth. Green plants, from lowly grass to lofty trees, together with water, hold the key to life on earth. Even the oceans contain many green plants.

The plant kingdom is a vast reservoir of energy. Plant foods capture the sun's rays and convert their energies into foods for man and beast. Animals cannot convert the energies that are in sun rays directly into energy that can be utilized by the body. The chlorophyll in the leaves of green plants converts sunlight into chemical energy, and we receive this chemical energy when we eat raw plant foods. All animals, including humans, depend on plants to do this for them.

The different wavelengths, or energies, of the sun's electromagnetic energy spectrum are believed to be one of the reasons there are so many different varieties of plants on the earth. It is believed that some plants are more receptive or attuned than others to the different wavelengths. Nutritionists tell us that the more varieties of plant foods we eat, the more we benefit from the different energies.

Raw plant foods are the unaltered and untainted foods as found in nature. They possess natural life force that enables the body to heal itself of diseases and other health disorders. The life force comes from the sun and is converted by plants into energy that humans and animals can utilize. When we eat raw (uncooked) fruits and vegetables, including green leafy vegetables, we get the precious life force that God intended for us to receive.

Raw plant foods possess the highest level of nutrients found in any food, and bestow numerous health benefits, some of which are yet to be discussed in this book. An abundance of vitality is available to anyone who adopts the raw vegan diet.

"Uncooked foods will supply not only all the necessary vitamins and minerals, but also all the enzymes and easily digestible natural starches and proteins needed for healthy functioning of the body." - Paavo O. Airola, N.D., *There is a Cure for Arthritis*.

On the raw vegan diet, the body's self-healing process operates most efficiently to purify the body of toxins and waste material. It is the body's self-cleansing process that enables us to heal ourselves of sickness and disease.

Cooked foods produce offensive wastes, most noticeable by the gas released during their digestion and the odor of the feces. The odor is also noticeable in the breath. These wastes gradually impair all the tissues and organs of the body, resulting in sickness and disease.

Raw plant foods are easier to digest than cooked foods, and leave fewer waste products behind. They do not cause offensive odors. They strengthen the entire organism in every respect because of the natural life force essence that is in them.

The high cost of health care in this country is linked in large part to the ill-health caused by eating foods that are harmful to the body. The increased supply of these foods has caused the deforestation of large parts of the earth in order to grow crops for animal feed.

The crops are needed to supply the ever-increasing number of Concentrated Animal Feeding Operations (CAFOs) that keep springing up everywhere. The proliferation of these animal-factories, with their huge demands for feed, water, and fossil-fuel energy, has created the need for GMO crops, together with their deadly pesticides and herbicides which are mainly responsible for the on-going extinction of the world's bee population, as well as causing health problems in people.

Every day we witness the affects that these foods have on us. It is no secret that sickness and disease continue to plague us despite the billions of dollars of federal, state and private funds spent each year trying to find cures for our diseases, including heart disease, cancer and the many other life-shortening and disabling diseases. Almost everyone knows someone who is suffering from a health issue. Most of us have come to accept sickness and disease as a normal part of life. But nutritionists have been telling us for years that these things do not happen by chance, but are caused by the foods we eat.

It is no coincidence that urgent care centers in this country have become as numerous and widespread as fast-food restaurants.

Raw plant foods have a benign and beneficial effect on the entire organism. After eating raw plant foods exclusively for only a short time, the body ramps up its self-cleansing process and focuses more on healing. Raw foodists throughout the world have been cleansed and healed of their health disorders by the powers of raw plant foods. These powers are made available to anyone who adopts a whole plant food diet such as the raw vegan diet.

The Bible describes not only what kind of foods we should eat but also their quantity. During their wilderness journeys, the children of Israel ate manna for 40 years before coming into the promised land. As stated in Exodus Chapter 16, each person was to eat no more than an omer of manna per day. An omer is an ancient unit of volume measurement equal to about 2 quarts. According to the Bible, it is best for us to eat no more than 2 quarts of food per day.

True health, which is health in tune with Nature, is gained when we adopt a whole plant food diet and reduce the quantity of the foods eaten. It is then that the body's self-healing process is fully engaged to produce true health. When true health arrives, it is like a sunrise after a long night, the kind of health you may never have experienced before.

Healthy people, healthy animals and healthy plants do not get sick. But health is not to be had for the asking. If it were, then everyone would be extraordinarily healthy. Rather, it must be gained. Food habits must be changed for the body to rid itself of the causes of ill-health, and to sustain itself in health.

The terms "God-given diet" and "raw vegan diet" will be used interchangeably in this book.

The Foods We Should Eat and Why

"He who does not know food, how can he understand the diseases of man?" - Hippocrates.

Much of what has been discussed in previous chapters provided reasons for avoiding certain types of foods and eating the right foods. This chapter explains more specifically what foods we should eat and why.

Increasing scientific evidence compiled every year links the top 10 leading causes of death, and the degenerative diseases so prevalent in the world today, to eating meat-based and dairy-based diets. These studies continue to show that people eating a plant-based diet have increased longevity and health compared to those eating a meat-based and/or dairy-based diet. Many books published in recent years provide the results of these clinical studies.

The China Study, published in 2005, may be the most comprehensive study of human nutrition ever performed. The population, or group, that was used in the study was the entire population of China. Written by T. Colin Campbell, a professor of Nutritional Biochemistry at Cornell University, and his son Thomas M. Campbell II, a physician, the study proved that whole plant-based foods, not animal-based foods, are the most beneficial foods for people. The study showed that people eating a plant-based diet have increased longevity and health compared to those eating a meat-based and/or dairy-based diet.

How Not to Die, written by Dr. Michael Greger and published in 2015, confirmed the conclusions of *The China Study*, and provided additional research and study results that emphasized the importance of eating plenty of whole plant foods, such as fruits and vegetables, to prevent and even reverse the chronic diseases of the Western world, including cancer, diabetes, heart disease and brain diseases.

The hazards of eating animal-based foods, or animal products, are well known to most educated people. Eating animal products causes plaque formations in the arteries, which is known to cause hardening of the arteries, which can lead to heart disease and stroke. Harmful mutagens and carcinogens, such as acrylamide, HCAs, PAHs and AGEs, are formed when animal products are cooked (for more detail, see Victoria Boutenko's book, *12 Steps to Raw Foods*). Animal products can contain nitrates, chlorine and ammonia and are susceptible to hosting various forms of life-destroying bacteria.

Studies conducted on animals and people show that blood cholesterol levels increase when animal protein is eaten. Dr. Caldwell Esselstyn, Jr., in his book, *Prevent and Reverse Heart Disease,* says that anyone with high blood cholesterol levels is prone to heart disease. Animal-based foods contain cholesterol, whereas no plant foods contain cholesterol. Dr. Esselstyn changed his diet to a plant-based diet and strongly recommended his patients to do the same. Those who did were able to cleanse their coronary arteries of plaque formations, which means their arteries were no longer clogged, and Dr. Esselstyn proved this by way of coronary angiograms.

Dr. Esselstyn is now a leading advocate of raw plant foods. He is featured in the food documentary DVD, *Forks Over Knives.* Testimonies given in that DVD attest to the powers of raw plant foods to heal a number of leading chronic diseases, including heart disease and breast cancer.

A Christian Diet

In *Fruits and Farinacea -- The Proper Food of Man*, John Smith tells us that based on all accessible sources, our progenitors were frugivorous, i.e., fruit eaters. Both anthropological studies and studies of how the human body functions support this conclusion.

"Meat is not man's natural food, since he is not either a carnivorous or an omnivorous animal. Every argument drawn from comparative anatomy, from physiology, from chemistry, from experience, from observation, and, when rightly used, from common sense, all agree that man is not a meat-eating animal. He can never be as healthy under the prevailing "mixed" diet as he would if he were to follow the dictates of Nature and live on his natural food – fruits and nuts, eaten in their uncooked, primitive form. Every element the system needs can be shown to be present in these foods, in their proper proportion, while, being live foods instead of mere "dead ashes", which is all the cooking process leaves, they will be found to supply a degree of vital life and energy which no cooked foods ever supplied or could supply."
- Hereward Carrington, *Vitality, Fasting and Nutrition.*

Human beings, in many key physiological ways, are not like other animals. We have hands with opposable thumbs, non-claw-like nails, teeth that are not suitable for tearing hide or flesh, or breaking bones, but rather for grinding plant foods, and long, not short, digestive tracts including 20-30 foot long intestines that are ideally suited for digesting fiber-rich foods like fruits, vegetables, nuts, seeds and grains.

David Wolfe in his book, The Sunfood Diet Success System, includes as Appendix A, an "Anatomy Chart" that identifies 17 physiological ways in which human beings are ideally suited for eating a plant-based diet. Websites also support this conclusion, as can be seen by searching on "are humans frugivores?"

These studies show that humans are naturally suited for picking, chewing and digesting plant-based foods. Chimpanzees, which are very similar to humans physiologically, subsist almost entirely on fruits and greens.

According to the Bible, the first people on earth lived to very great ages. Adam lived to 930 years   Methuselah lived 969 years. Prior to the Flood, the average human lifespan was about 900 years. However, immediately after the Flood, when animal food was permitted to be eaten, the average lifespan fell to about 400 years. Later, when Jacob, the father of the twelve tribes of Israel, lived, the average lifespan was only about 150 years.

Based on the latest worldwide statistics from WHO, the average human lifespan is currently 72 years.

The worldwide increase in food production has resulted in a worldwide topsoil mineral deficiency. The topsoil in which plants are grown is now depleted of its minerals. Reports on the Web cover recent losses of nutrients in crops. Only decades ago, the same crops were richer in vitamins and minerals. Meat and dairy products (animal products) are affected even worse. Animals consume the mineral deficient crops and become mineral deficient. Cooking animal products further depletes them of minerals and vitamins.

The mineral deficiency of the topsoil is being blamed on improper farm management practices resulting in ill-replenishment of the minerals back into the soil. The meteoric rise in food productivity and efficiency since the last century have not been balanced by a corresponding increase in the addition of nutrients back into the soil.

Nutritional deficiency occurs when the body does not absorb or get enough of the necessary amounts of nutrients it needs from foods. Nutrients include vitamins, minerals, proteins, carbohydrates, fats and water. They are essential for cellular growth and the maintenance of life. The body does not manufacture nutrients, but obtains them from the surrounding environment. We get most of our nutrients from foods.

People who eat the traditional American diet are nutrient deficient. This deficiency has been shown to be the cause of a number of serious health problems. To make up for the mineral-starved and vitamin-starved foods now being produced, many people take multivitamin/mineral supplements on the advice of their doctors. According to the Web, billions of dollars are spent each year in America alone on these supplements.

Unfortunately, most of the multivitamin/mineral supplements are inorganic substances that cannot be utilized by the body. Studies have shown that these supplements provide little, if any, benefit to human health. See Web articles, such as from searching on "multivitamin/mineral supplements." It is also discussed in books by Dr. Ann Wigmore (see Bibliography), among others.

"Inorganic minerals are rejected by the cells of the body, which, if not evacuated, can cause arterial obstructions and even more serious damage." - Norman W. Walker, *Water Can Undermine Your Health.*

According to many nutritionists who are referenced in this book, the cells of the body can only utilize minerals that are in organic form, which is one of the reasons why plant foods are so important to us. Plants convert inorganic minerals found in the soil and water into organic form that is readily assimilated by the cells of the body.

A Christian Diet

Doctors often prescribe medication that is calcium carbonate based, which an inorganic mineral compound. Calcium carbonate is the main ingredient in almost all antacids, and it is also found in some brands of aspirin.

The days when milk cows roamed the pastures and got their calcium from grass are over. Today's milk cows do not go outside to graze. They seldom move out of their stalls or feedlots. Their urine and feces are removed mechanically. Their milk is removed by machines hooked up to their udders. They get their calcium and other nutrients from their feed, which, according to Web articles, is a specially formulated mix of grains, soy, silage and inorganic calcium in the form of calcite flour (calcium carbonate), aragonite (calcium carbonate), crushed bones, and other bits and pieces of slaughtered animals to maximize weight gain and therefore profits when the cows are no longer useful as money-making machines. Apparently, calcium from cow's milk is mainly inorganic calcium.

On the raw vegan diet, there is no need for multivitamin/mineral supplements, since all the minerals and vitamins needed to support life are in raw plant foods in their proper organic form and undestroyed by heat. An example is the amount of organic calcium that is in collard greens. According to the USDA publication Nutritive Value of American Foods, just two-thirds cup of collard greens has 91% of the calcium in a cup of milk. Other plant foods having about the same amount of calcium are kelp and almonds.

A whole plant food diet also compensates for topsoil mineral deficiency since more plant foods are eaten on the diet. In addition, the diet includes sea vegetables, which are grown in the ocean -- a mineral-rich environment.

Nutritional deficiency is so widespread in this country and in the world today that it can be said to be the number one health problem in the world, even among people who supposedly eat a healthy, balanced diet.

Excitotoxins are substances added to processed foods and beverages for the purpose of stimulating brain neurons. For years, the food industry has designed food products to titillate the taste buds and activate the reward centers of the brain. The diverse chemicals that are used for these purposes include excitotoxins. The term was popularized by Dr. Russel Blaylock in his book, *Excitotoxins, The Taste that Kills*. As stated in the book, these substances are found in almost all processed foods. Excitotoxins include monosodium glutamate (MSG)[5], aspartame (used in artificial sweeteners), cysteine (used in breads), hydrolyzed protein, and aspartic acid. These substances can stimulate brain neurons so severely that they are killed, resulting in varying degrees of brain damage.

Remember that piercing headache you got the last time you ate Chinese food? It was probably due to the MSG used on the food. The Web adequately covers the dangers of MSG, e.g., do a search on "msg in foods."

As of this writing, there are no regulations requiring the food industry to test its products for whether they cause brain damage or food addictions.

The deliberate tampering of foods to increase taste appeal at the expense of harming the body, while attesting to the inventiveness

---

[5] According to Blaylock's book, the food industry is on a quest to disguise MSG in foods. A list of common additives that contain MSG is found in the book.

and ingenuity of the American spirit, typifies how low we have sunk in manipulating foods for financial gain.

It is entirely possible that the causative factor, or at least a major contributing factor, to the sharp rise in brain diseases in our culture, including dementia and other neurological disorders, is the continued use year after year of food products that contain excitotoxins. I recommend Dr. Blaylock's book to anyone. It includes a list of chemicals that should be tacked to our kitchen walls. It will make you check the foods labels all over again.

To avoid the hazards that have been described, and more (I'm sure I haven't mentioned all of them) we should eat raw plant foods. This is what nutritional experts have been telling us for years, as documented in their books listed in the Bibliography.

We live in the age of information, and the Web/Internet is our most popular information source. While I consider the Web a very useful tool for learning about foods and nutrition, it should not be our only source for this information. Much of what is on websites is opinion-oriented or provided in support of commercial interests. Opinions can run the gamut, and misrepresentation and conflicting information can be, and often times are, the result.

"As corrupting an influence as money is in medicine, it appears to be even worse in the field of nutrition, where it seems everyone has his or her own brand of snake oil supplement or wonder gadget. Dogmas are entrenched and data too often cherry picked to support preconceived notions." - Dr. Michael Greger, *How Not To Die*.

For example, for years leading nutritionists have contended that cooked and starchy foods are detrimental to human health, and that abstinence from such foods is necessary to cure health disorders including diseases. However, at the time of this writing, many of the websites queried for this information actually *encourage* eating cooked and starchy foods as part of a healthy diet.

We cannot trust everything we read on the Web. But that being said, the Web should not be ignored as a learning tool in self-education about foods and nutrition. However, for those of us who are seeking answers to the really tough questions of today about foods and nutrition, books provide the answers. The books that are listed in the Bibliography are excellent resources that will aid anyone in their quest for a more thorough understanding of foods and nutrition.

Books have the answers on how to gain optimum health, the Web does not. Books cannot be easily condensed into Web articles, and typically provide comprehensive coverage of the issues, or they refer to other books or studies that provide the information. In addition, books are typically written by competent and knowledgeable authors who provide good, proven advice.

Today's real need is not another low-carb, high-protein diet, or an end to global warming, which appears to be mainly caused by extensive deforestation efforts to clear space for cattle and feed crops. Rather, it is self-education about foods and nutrition.

Typically, people resort to doctors when they don't know what else to do. But by simply utilizing the Web/Internet, as well as the information that is contained in books that are available to most people, many health concerns can be thoroughly investigated, and the proper treatments determined, without seeing a physician.

The body can take a lot of punishment and abuse. It can survive both drought and famine. It can live on junk food for decades without showing many ill effects. But the body does not thrive on drought or famine or junk food. It thrives on life-giving plant foods. If optimum health is the goal, then a change in the diet is required.

None of us has to die of a disease caused by eating a bad diet, and none of us has to endure the many attendant complications and discomforts of a disease prior to death. And we won't, if we take care of our bodies by giving it the life-giving foods it needs.

It is our responsibility to take care of our bodies. It is not our doctor's, our spouse's, our friends' or the Government's. It is our responsibility. We should avoid foods that are harmful to health and eat foods that promote health and longevity. These are whole plant foods, replete with their life-giving properties. These are the foods that God and Nature intended for us to eat.

"But the foods which you eat from the abundant table of God give you strength and youth to your body, and you will never see disease. For the table of God fed Methuselah of old, and I tell you truly, if you live as he lived, then will the God of the living give you also long life upon the earth as was his." - Attributed to Jesus, *The Essene Gospel of Peace, Book One.*

• *Fruits and Vegetables*

Raw fruits and vegetables are eaten regularly on the raw vegan diet, for good reasons. They digest easily and efficiently because their enzymes have not been destroyed by heat. Enzymes have life force properties that Nature intended for us to receive, that support all bodily functions and contain the vitamins and nutrients the body needs for optimum health. (Note: enzymes are further discussed in the chapter on "The Dangers of Cooked Foods.")

Fruits and vegetables are best eaten when they are ripe. If eaten in their typical store-bought, un-ripened condition, stomachache or some other discomfort is likely. Also, extra energy is required to digest them, and this energy is taken from the energy reserves of the body when it could be used for other purposes, such as healing and self-cleansing.

Fruits and vegetables sold at local food stores are typically shipped-in from distant locations, such as foreign countries, and purposely arrive in an un-ripened condition in order to retard spoilage and prolong shelf-life. To ripen store-bought fruits and vegetables, just set them on the counter tops at home until they are ripe; it usually takes several days, depending on the fruit or vegetable. For example, bananas are typically sold green or partly green in color, unless you happen by the fruit stand right before the bananas are replaced. Ripe bananas are speckled or streaked brown in color, which typically takes several days.

Cucumbers are ripe when they are easily flexed. Avocados are ripe when they yield to gentle pressure. Green chilies and jalapenos are ripe when they turn orange or red, do not eat them when they are green. Lemons, limes, oranges and pears are ripe when they are aromatic. Same for red and yellow peppers.

Some exceptions to this are apples (all varieties) and root vegetables (e.g., carrots, beets, turnips, radishes, potatoes, onions, garlic, etc.). Apples and root vegetables do not ripen to any significant extent after they are picked.

Fruits are nutritious and stimulating, and have many healing qualities. They act to cleanse and energize the cells of the body. I consider fruits to be the ideal food for humankind.

"Fruits alone, even of but one kind, not only heal but nourish perfectly the human body, eliminating entirely the possibility of disease." - Arnold Ehret, *Mucusless Diet Healing System*.

Some people will not eat fruit because the last time they did, it caused them too much discomfort. Most likely, it was because the fruit was eaten in an un-ripened condition, or else it was combined improperly with other foods. For example, when dates or figs are eaten with pineapple, the result may be a stomachache, because sweet fruit (dates and figs) should not be eaten with acid fruit (pineapple). See the chapter on "Proper Food Combinations."

The importance of eating fruit on the raw vegan diet cannot be overemphasized, and will be discussed further in this book.

Fatty fruits include avocados and olives. They contain healthy unsaturated fat. Some nutritional experts consider avocado a Superfood, although it is not classified as such. Superfoods have super high-density nutritional value (see subsection on Superfoods). The avocado contains a substantial amount of monounsaturated fats, phytosterols and antioxidants like vitamin E, vitamin C, and carotenoids. It is also high in beta-sitosterol (95 mg per medium-sized avocado) which is known to assist in relieving prostate disorders, such as benign prostatic hyperplasia (BPH).

Plain avocado can be used like butter on raw vegetables such as cabbage, broccoli, cucumber, cauliflower, carrots, asparagus, green onions, tomatoes, chili peppers and celery - with great results. Or, you can make an avocado-based dipping sauce, such as the one described below. But it's mainly fat, so use avocado in moderation.

The vegetables that have the most tightly compacted layers are some of the most nutritious. They include red and green cabbage, leeks, broccoli, bok choy, green onions, lettuce and celery.

Carrots are high in beta-carotene which is converted to vitamin A in the body. The word "carotene" is derived from the Latin word for carrot, "carota." Nutritional expert N.W. Walker in his books (see Bibliography), states that raw carrots have all the elements and vitamins that are required by the human body. It could just be that the "lowly carrot" is capable of making up for many of the nutritional deficiencies in the world today.

Carrots are non-starchy vegetables (see the chapter on "Proper Food Combinations").

Red beets are good for the blood. They lower blood pressure. They improve athletic performance. They are one of the highest of oxygenating foods. Marathon runners are partial to them because they increase their endurance. After consuming red beets, it takes less energy to run a race. This makes red beets important for elderly health, since studies have shown that there is a decline in maximal oxygen consumption with age. In addition, red beets have a high acid-binding rating (see Berg's Tables in the Appendix).

I haven't forgotten about leafy greens, which are one of the most important foods we can eat on the raw vegan diet. I consider them their own food group as will be discussed soon.

A Vegetable Dipping Sauce

A meal that makes you sit straight up in a chair is a tasty meal. Raw plant foods do not have to be boring, bland affairs. They can be tasty meals, and, for effective digestion, the mouth should water before and during a meal.

There are plenty of nutritious raw plant food recipes in well-thought-out raw food recipe books, such as Kristina Carrillo-Bucaram's book, *The Fully Raw Diet.*

I would avoid using raw food recipes on the Web, since they often combine fruits and vegetables improperly. No one needs to turn a meal into a gastronomic catastrophe. Meals should be tasty, but they should go easy on the stomach.

The following dipping sauce makes all vegetables and greens more palatable. While intended for those just starting out on a whole plant food diet, it can be used with great success also by experienced raw food eaters. It is the only recipe in this book.

How to Make the Sauce:

• Prepare several large avocados, sans skins, in a large bowl or container.
• Blend (using a blender) a few large carrots and/or red beets in water, and then add them to the avocados.
• Blend 5 lemons, 5 garlic cloves, and 1 skinned red or yellow onion (or 2 bunches of green onions) in water, and add to the mixture.
• Add unrefined, natural sea salt to taste (for the benefits of using natural sea salt, see the chapter on "The Good and Bad About Salt").

The sauce has six important tastes to stimulate the corresponding six groups of taste buds -- sour (lemons), spicy (garlic), bitter (onions), fat (avocado), sweet (all vegetables contain natural sugars) and salty. It makes rainbow kale or broccoli sprouts a complete meal, and enhances the taste of all other vegetables.

No short cuts! A mistake that raw food eaters sometimes make is taking short cuts. If lemon or lime juice from 100% concentrate is used in the above dipping sauce recipe, we are adding cooked foods because juice from 100% concentrate is a pasteurized, processed food product. If you are faithful to the raw vegan diet, you will reap the full benefits of the diet.

No fruit or vegetable is intrinsically better than another. Each may be preferred, or not, depending on a person's nutritional needs and personal preferences. We all have grown to like certain fruits or vegetables better than others, and we all have slightly different nutritional needs. The only way to learn what fruits and vegetables are best for us, is to eat a variety of them in their ripened states, and, if not by themselves in mono meals, then ensuring that they are eaten properly combined with other foods.

David Wolfe states in one of his books that there are so many edible fruits and vegetables in the world that if you tried a new kind every day of your life, you would never live long enough to try them all. So, what is stopping us from trying the 40-50 varieties of fruits and vegetables that are in our local food stores? It's the only way to know whether they work for us nutritionally and otherwise.

Grains and Legumes

Technically speaking, grains are seeds of grasses. However, they are commonly considered to be vegetables. Grains include wheat, corn, oats, barley, rye, millet, and rice. Grain products include refined flour products, such as white bread, cereal, white and brown rice and pasta.

Most grains are starchy foods. For that reason, I no longer eat grains, nor do I advise their use on the raw vegan diet. If you eat grains, they should be kept to a minimum part of the diet. Many nutritionists believe that eating these foods leads to constipation and then to disease. More about this is provided in the chapter on "The Dangers of Starchy Foods."

Legumes include peas, beans, peanuts and lentils. Legumes are commonly considered to be vegetables. Like grains, they are starchy foods, and for that reason I no longer eat them, nor do I advise their use on the raw vegan diet.

• *Greens (Leafy Green Vegetables)*

Leafy greens are commonly considered vegetables, but I agree with Victoria Boutenko in her book, *Green for Life*, that greens should be their own food group. Greens are the only foods that combine well with all other foods, including other greens. You can't say that about many fruits and vegetables or nuts and seeds.

Leafy greens include spinach, arugula, chard, kale (several varieties), mustard greens, collard greens, turnip greens, parsley, cilantro, lettuce (several varieties), celery greens and dandelion.

A good way to add greens to our diet is to drink green smoothies. They provide the health benefits of fruits and greens in a single meal. Try apricots, bananas, lemons, mangos (in season) with kale, spinach, romaine lettuce, or chard. Watch the way you combine fruits to ensure adherence to the food combination laws, which are discussed in the chapter on "Proper Food Combinations." You should rotate the greens every week or so to avoid alkaloid buildup, which is caused when too much of one kind of greens are eaten.

The chlorophyll in greens strengthens the immune system, helps to detoxify the body and improves digestion. Chlorophyll is rich in antioxidants, minerals, vitamins and readily assimilated enzymes. The chlorophyll in green plants is what converts sunlight into chemical energy, and this energy is made available to us when we eat greens.

Eating a variety of greens ensures that we receive all the amino acids we need in our diets. In his book, *The China Study*, T. Colin Campbell states that plant protein is the healthiest type of protein because it allows for slow but steady synthesis of the proteins.

"Greens are the primary food group that matches human nutritional needs most completely…Chlorophyll is liquefied sun energy. Consuming as much chlorophyll as possible is like bathing our inner organs in sunshine." - Victoria Boutenko, *Green for Life*.

Cilantro is high in potassium and vitamins A, B, C and K and has antifungal, antioxidant and antibacterial properties.

Women should eat more greens. It is known that menstruation difficulties or pains find their solution in eating greens. The importance of eating greens cannot be overemphasized, for the simple reason that few things in life are more important for health.

Store-bought arugula (shipped-in from elsewhere, not locally) is much milder than the arugula I get from my local Community Supported Agriculture (CSA) farm. The CSA arugula is noticeably spicier (more peppery), like mild chili peppers. What does this difference in taste mean? Studies have shown that foods grown locally and harvested recently are superior nutritionally to store-bought foods. You can taste the difference. The studies show that fruits and vegetables lose vitamins while in storage and transit. Lettuce loses about 50% of its key nutrients. For Web articles about this, e.g., search on "home grown vs. store bought produce."

The cost difference between organic and conventionally grown produce is typically only a matter of nickels and dimes, rather than dollars as it used to be. In my opinion, the advantages of organic foods far outweigh any small cost differential.

The Importance of Organic Foods

Federal regulations in the US stipulate that organic foods cannot be grown with synthetic (man-made) fertilizers, synthetic pesticides or sewage sludge. As such, organic foods do not contain harmful or potentially toxic substances. These regulations were a long time in coming.

Organic foods are not irradiated[6], and they are not GMO-modified (i.e., Genetically Modified Organisms). Organic produce will typically have the "USDA Organic" label, but may have the "CCOF (California Certified Organic Farmers) Organic" label which is somewhat less restrictive than the "USDA Organic" label. Other organizations are also USDA certified, such as Oregon Tilth, which uses the "Oregon Tilth Certified Organic" (OTCO) label.

There are now more certified organic growers/farmers in this country than ever before. Accordingly, prices have gone down for organic foods.

---

[6] Dr. Edward Howell states in his book, Enzyme Nutrition, that the use of radiation to preserve foods results in the wholesale destruction of all the enzymes and vital properties contained in the foods.

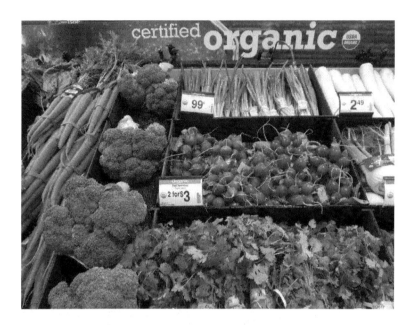

We can buy non-organic bananas, lemons, limes, pineapples, avocados, onions and garlic because they require less pesticides in their cultivation, so they should have less pesticide residues on them. Also, we don't usually eat the skins of these foods. In addition, they are non-GMO crops (see the chapter on "GMO Crops").

Pesticides

Pesticides are poisons that are sprayed on conventionally-grown plant foods in order to kill pests that attack the crops. USDA tests have shown that pesticide contamination levels on plant foods can vary depending on the crop and where it is grown.

If pesticides can kill other life forms, then they may also be injurious to human life. Studies have shown that pesticides are indeed injurious to human health. The dangers of pesticides are adequately covered on the Web, and in the books listed in the Bibliography.

Lists of fruits and vegetables that have the least and the most pesticides on them are provided on the Web. Two of these lists, the "Clean 15" and the "Dirty Dozen", are provided in Appendix II. However, a comment about these lists is in order. Not all fruits and vegetables are included in these lists. Also, the lists may not be completely reliable. For example, cabbage, which is one of my favorite vegetables, is listed in the "Clean 15" list, indicating that I can purchase it conventionally grown and do not have to buy it "organic."

However, according to David Wolfe's book, *The Sunfood Diet Success System*, large amounts of pesticides are used on non-organic cabbage. I searched the Web to confirm this but could not find the information of Wolfe's book on the Web. I wanted to be sure, so I ate non-organic white/green cabbage for a week. Small red, itchy sores erupted on my skin, and I'm not allergic to cabbage. I have the same reaction whenever I eat non-organic foods that have high pesticide residues. While this is not conclusive or scientific proof, it leads me to believe that cabbage should not be listed on the "Clean 15" list.

• *Nuts and Seeds*

To get our daily complement of saturated fats, nuts and seeds may be eaten. Nuts come from trees. The peanut, which is not really a nut but a legume, grows in the ground.

Nuts and seeds contain vitamins, minerals and folic acid which are needed by the body. However, many of the commercially available nuts and seeds are refined and processed foods that should not be eaten on the diet. They include the many roasted and salted varieties. The life force properties of these foods have been destroyed by heat. A roasted or pasteurized nut or seed planted in the ground will not grow.

I used to buy "raw almonds" from the local food stores. The labels clearly state "Raw Almonds." However, I learned that almonds are required by law (such as California State law) to be steam-pasteurized. The same goes for hazelnuts (filberts). Therefore, if we buy "raw" almonds or hazelnuts purchased from local food stores, the chances are we are buying pasteurized nuts with their enzymes destroyed. Pasteurized nuts have some nutritional value but they do not have the life force properties of raw plant foods, and should therefore be avoided on the diet.

Nuts and seeds easily absorb pesticides. Many are imported from distant countries, such as Africa, where food products may not be properly monitored or controlled for pesticide residues. Per the Web, peanuts, pistachios and cashews have the worst pesticide residues. Therefore, to minimize pesticides in your diet, buy raw, "organic" nuts and seeds. If you cannot find them at local food stores, they can be purchased from websites.

Nuts and seeds combine well with themselves and with most vegetables. Fatty nuts (like pecans) combine well with sweet fruits.

FAT VS PROTEIN CONTENT OF NUTS AND SEEDS (FAT / PROTEIN)

Almonds   2/1

Brazil Nuts   4/1

Cashews	2/1
Hazelnuts	4/1
Pecans	10/1
Pistachios	2/1
Walnuts	4/1
Pumpkin Seeds	1.5/1
Sunflower Seeds	3/1

As seen above, nuts and seeds are fat-dominant foods, not protein-dominant foods. David Wolfe, in *The Sunfood Diet Success System*, agrees. However, this is not reflected in many articles on the Web which claim that nuts and seeds are protein-dominant foods. More on this in the chapter on "Proper Food Combinations."

Sprouting

I believe that everyone on the raw vegan diet should learn how to sprout **foods. It puts you in the driver's seat and gives you complete control over what you eat.**

Sprouts are the initial forms of plants after they germinate from seeds. When a seed germinates, its life force is at a peak level. Eating sprouts is highly recommended for their abundant supply of enzymes and nutrients. Fully sprouted seeds, such as clover or broccoli sprouts, can be purchased from whole food stores. Whether purchased or home-grown, sprouts should be included in the raw vegan diet on a frequent basis.

Soaking raw nuts and seeds in water causes them to sprout. Some exceptions to this, however, are pecans, walnuts and Brazil nuts.

Basically, here's how to sprout nuts and seeds at home. Add raw (unpasteurized) nuts or seeds to a quart jar to about 1/2 full because they will expand when soaked, then fill with water and let them soak overnight. In the morning, drain the water and let them dry sufficiently. You can dry them at home in the kitchen, in the sun or you can use a dehydrator at about 115° F. Drying times can be several days or more. When they are thoroughly dry, then eat them and benefit from their abundant life force.

When I began sprouting, I read sprouting books, purchased the seeds, quart jars and wicker baskets, and learned the proper techniques. You can best learn how to grow your own sprouts at home by reading Dr. Ann Wigmore's book, *The Sprouting Book*, and Steve ("Sproutman") Meyerowitz's book, *Sprouts, The Miracle Food*.

Sprouting is a survival tactic that may be useful someday. The basics required are only seeds, water, air and a little sunshine. A person could live a long time on nothing but sprouts.

Sprouting can be messy and clutter up the kitchen, but that can be avoided or minimized by the sprouting method used. There are now some very inventive and easy to use DIY kits available on the Web for sprouting at home. In any case, the remarkable life force in sprouts outweighs any minor inconveniences.

• *Sea Vegetables*

"The composition of the human body and the composition of seven gallons of sea water are the same. In view of this fact, it would seem practical to turn to the sea in order to supply the nutrient needs of the body." - Dr. D. C. Jarvis, *Folk Medicine*.

Sea vegetables are important adjuncts to land vegetables in the raw vegan diet. As mentioned previously, the topsoil worldwide is minerally deficient. Sea vegetables obtain their minerals from the ocean, which is a mineral-rich environment and practically unaffected by topsoil mineral deficiency.

Sea vegetables, including kelp and dulse, are our main source of iodine. Sea vegetables are also high in potassium. Both of these minerals are often lacking in today's land-grown crops. Iodine is needed for the proper functioning of the thyroid gland and potassium is needed for the proper functioning of the nervous system.

While natural sea salt contains iodine from the sea, it provides less of what we need daily. Nutritional experts such as Dr. D. C. Jarvis, recommend taking 1/4 to 1/2 teaspoons of kelp or dulse per day to meet the daily iodine requirement.

"There is a definite relationship between the amount of energy you have and your iodine intake." - Dr. D. C. Jarvis, *Folk Medicine*.

According to Dr. Bernard Jensen in his book, *Guide to Diet and Detoxification,* dulse may be the best source of iodine because it contains more manganese which assists in the absorption of iodine in the body. Kelp and dulse are available in powder, tablet and liquid form.

When I was macrobiotic years ago, I ate brown rice balls with nori, a sea vegetable. When I switched to a vegetarian diet with fish, I stopped eating nori. I now eat sea vegetables almost daily and have experienced their benefits.

However, do not discount the possibility that your tastes and food choices will change with time on the raw vegan diet.

• *Superfoods*

Superfoods are the foods of the future in the sense that many people are not familiar with them. David Wolfe in his book, Superfoods, defines them as: "plant foods with super high-density nutritional value."

In my opinion, Superfoods should be added cautiously to the diet because of their potency and unique characteristics. The road to Superfoods turns into some very exciting country, but go slow, there are some hazards.

I recommend adding only one Superfood at a time to the diet, so that each may be tested to see what they do for you, or against you. That way you avoid the pitfalls of eating Superfoods together and possibly violating food combination laws, and also, you'll be better able to utilize the knowledge gained about each Superfood when it is advantageous for you to do so.

The following Superfoods are discussed herein.

• Aloe Vera

• Spirulina

• Hemp Seed

• Goji Berries

• Bee Products

- Cacao Beans

- Maca

- Coconut

There are more Superfoods than those listed, but those discussed are the most commonly eaten on the raw vegan diet. For more Superfood information, see David Wolfe's book, *Superfoods*.

Aloe Vera

Aloe Vera is a medium-sized, green and firm-leaf plant with leaves consisting of a gelatinous interior surrounded by a skin with thorns on the edges of the leaves. It is rich in antioxidants, amino acids and enzymes that help cleanse the body of toxins. It is well known to have curative powers for healing cuts and burns. You don't have to de-skin the leaves or cut off the thorns; each leaf can be eaten raw. Aloe Vera, like chayote, has very little aroma until it is cut into.

Like the palm tree, it grows without much assistance in sunny climates. To eat Aloe Vera, cut off the lower leaves which are the first to droop and die. If the leaves are stored in the refrigerator, they last for weeks. After a few days of storage, the thorns are soft enough to eat, so you don't have to remove them.

Eating more than a small amount of Aloe Vera leaf per day may cause gas or other complications. Aloe Vera is a very effective bowel cleanser.

Spirulina

Spirulina is a blue-green fresh water algae. It is typically grown in lakes. It is lauded for its amazing health benefits. It is high in protein, and contains antioxidants, B-complex vitamins, beta-carotene, vitamin E, manganese, zinc, copper, iron, selenium, and gamma linolenic acid. It is one of the few plant sources of the DHA/EPA and ALA omega-3 fatty acids, the other being chlorella.

Spirulina is about 50% protein by weight, making it one of the highest protein plant foods available. On the raw vegan diet, it is easy to get all the protein you need from leafy greens and vegetables, but if you're worried about not getting enough protein, then add spirulina to your next meal. However, watch how you combine it with other foods.

Spirulina is typically sold in powdered form which is easily added to anything.

Despite its many benefits, I have found that spirulina causes very foul-smelling gas. Spirulina is a form of bacteria, of the phylum Cyanobacteria. When it gets into the intestines it can cause friendly bacteria to proliferate to an extent that causes excess gas.

Chlorella, also considered a superfood, is similar to spirulina and also causes smelly gas, at least for me. For that reason, I no longer use these products.

Hemp Seed

Hemp Seed is said to be the most nutritious seed in the world. It contains all the essential amino acids and fatty acids that are required for human life. It is high in protein (but not as much as spirulina – see table below), antioxidants, iron, zinc, carotene, phytosterols, vitamins and enzymes. Hemp seeds have an ideal ratio of omega 6 to omega 3 fatty acids, and because of this they are preferred over flaxseeds and chia seeds for omega 3.

When I first tried hemp seeds, I was surprised that they were not hard seeds like many other seeds. They are soft seeds and have a mild, nutty, or grain-like flavor.

Goji Berries

Goji berries, which are native to China, are bright-red berries that grow on shrubs. They are high in antioxidants and nutrients. They make an excellent snack food when eaten by themselves. However, when combined with other foods, except for greens, the combinations should adhere to the food combination laws (see chapter on Proper Food Combinations).

Contrary to articles on the Web which indicate that goji berries combine well with sweet fruit, such as raisons, and also with protein foods, such as nuts, seeds and hemp seed, as in trail mix, I discovered it was not the case. Such food combinations cause stomachaches indicative of not adhering to the laws of nature that include the rules of proper food combining.

Almost all goji berries sold on the market today are of the dried fruit kind. They look, feel and taste like raisins. But unlike raisins, which are sweet fruit, goji berries, in my opinion, are acid or sub-acid fruit. They combine well with pineapple, cherries and raspberries, but do not combine well with sweet fruit, such as figs or grapes, or with protein foods, such as nuts and seeds.

Goji berries have the peculiar distinction of being adaptogens, which are substances that exert a normalizing effect on bodily processes. Ginseng is a well-known example.

I first purchased goji berries from local whole foods stores, but later found better prices on the Web.

Bee Products[7]

Bee product superfoods include honey, bee pollen and royal jelly. Another bee product, honeycomb, is not considered a superfood.

Honey is made by bees from the nectar of flowers and plants that bees visit when pollenating them. Raw honey contains many minerals, amino acids and enzymes.

Most of the honey consumed today is refined honey, which is pasteurized so its enzymes have been destroyed. If the label does not say "raw," then it is refined and processed honey.

Dr. D. C. Jarvis in his book, *Arthritis and Folk Medicine*, states that the nutritional value of foods is improved by the ability of honey to extract from the foods what the body needs. He also states that it has been the experience of generations of Vermonters that beekeepers do not have kidney trouble, and do not develop cancer or paralysis.

---

[7] Bee products are often contested as not being raw vegan food since they come from bees, which are animals. However, there are many nutritionists, among them Ann Wigmore, Norman W. Walker, Herbert M. Shelton and David Wolf, who advocate including bee products in the raw vegan diet. In my opinion, this issue is, in the overall picture of things, a minor point of contestability, especially when the health benefits of bee products are considered. In any case, each of us must decide how we stand on this issue. Like any other types of food, if bee products do not work for you, then they should be avoided.

David Wolfe in his book, *Superfoods*, states that bee pollen is the most complete Superfood there is. Royal jelly, another bee product, is what bees feed to the larvae in the hive. It is also highly nutritious.

Unfortunately, the worldwide population of bees is declining. The on-going extinction is blamed on the widespread use of pesticides on crops. This has the potential of adversely affecting all of us. If it is not turned around soon, it will have dire consequences for the pollination of plants, which means the production of fruits and all other plants that require pollination for their reproduction. This tragedy is documented in Horst Kornberger's book, *Global Hive: Bee Crisis and Compassionate Ecology*. The Web adequately covers this issue. It is also covered in some DVDs that are available on the subject.

Organic, raw, unfiltered honey has not been adulterated in any way and is the best honey to eat for health benefits. You can squeeze honey on salads, add unrefined sea salt and some water, and it tastes like French dressing. Or add it to apple cider vinegar to make a cure all drink that has been used for centuries in the US to cure many human ailments (see the last section of this chapter).

Cacao Beans

Cacao beans are not really beans (legumes) but the seeds of the cacao tree.

Cacao beans are very high in antioxidants and nutrients. Crushed cacao beans are called cacao nibs. Cacao nibs have been dried and fermented but are apparently the least processed of the available forms of chocolate. If you want to try a more natural form chocolate, then cacao nibs are the product to buy. Cacao nibs are crunchy and have a slightly bitter taste. Soaking cacao nibs in water makes them softer and easier to chew.

There are two powdered forms of the cacao bean: 1) cacao powder and 2) cocoa powder. They are similar but not the same thing. They taste the same, but taste is often deceiving. Both cacao powder and cocoa powder are refined and processed foods, but cacao powder is the least refined form. Cacao powder is made by cold-pressing unroasted cacao beans. It is claimed that the cold-pressing process does not destroy any of the bean's enzymes and nutrients. Cocoa powder is made by roasting the cacao beans.

A useful yardstick of food value is Oxygen Radical Absorbance Capacity (ORAC), which is an antioxidant rating that was used by the USDA until 2012. It is still used as a comparative basis for antioxidant capacity. Per the Web, the ORAC value of raw cacao powder is 95,500, which is the highest rating of all forms of chocolate. The ORAC value of roasted cocoa powder is 26,000. More about ORAC in the chapter on "Antioxidants."

Everyone likes chocolate, but have you tried the genuine article, cacao nibs?

Maca

Maca, like goji berries, is also an adaptogen. Maca is known to increase energy levels and enhance libido. Some claim that it is an aphrodisiac. It is typically sold in powdered form, which is easily added to anything.

Maca has a butterscotch color and a mild, butterscotch flavor. When I first tried it, I combined it with spirulina in my vegetable dipping sauce. This resulted in violating a food combination law and caused me to have a big stomachache. Maca is a starchy food, whereas spirulina is a protein food. Starchy foods and protein foods should not be eaten together (see the chapter on "Proper Food Combinations"). However, when properly combined with other foods, Maca adds real gusto to life. When I combined it properly, I was impressed by the increase in energy I experienced.

Maca is also available in a near starch-free powder, called Gelatinized Maca, but the product undergoes additional refining and does not have the life force properties of regular Maca.

In my opinion, Maca is a very powerful Superfood. We don't understand all of its benefits, but it should be used moderately.

Maca is 32% starch (see the chapter on "Proper Food Combinations"). It is, therefore, a starchy food. I no longer eat Maca because I no longer eat starchy foods (see the chapter on "The Dangers of Starchy Foods").

Coconut

Coconut provides health benefits, such as protecting against heart disease and stroke, and has the capability to neutralize or eradicate Candida and other pathogenic microorganisms. It is tasty by itself or when combined with chocolate (cacao beans), and it also makes a great addition to green smoothies.

Coconut is about one-third saturated fat. The saturated fat in coconut is a healthy saturated fat, which is different from the saturated fat found in animal products. The saturated fat in coconut is a medium-chain fatty acid that is easily assimilated by the body. The saturated fat in animal products is a long-chain fatty acid that is difficult to assimilate by the body. Coconut does not contribute to blood cholesterol levels as opposed to the long-chain fatty acids that are found in animal products.[8]

To open a coconut, the recommended approach is to wrap it in a towel and hit it with a hammer. I use a plastic grocery bag instead of a towel for easier clean up. The Web may be useful here. It has YouTube videos on how to open and peel coconuts. You can drop them on the floor to crack them open. Then, pry the shell apart with a large knife, and separate the meat from the shell using a knife or other tool. The meat can be frozen for later use.

The protein content of selected raw plant foods is given below, compiled from books in the Bibliography and from Web articles. Some may find it useful for ensuring adherence to the food combination laws, and it should dampen the fears of those who are worried about not getting enough protein on the raw vegan diet.

PROTEIN CONTENT OF RAW PLANT FOODS

Spirulina	50%
Hemp Seeds	30%
Pumpkin Seeds	28%
Pistachios	20%
Sesame Seeds	20%

---

[8] Coconut oil, the kind typically sold in bottles, is a fractionated oil that is known to raise cholesterol levels in people, per Victoria Boutenko's book, Raw & Beyond. Fractionated oils also include other so-called "healthy" oils, such as olive oil and avocado oil. It is best to stay away from oils.

Cacao Beans	20%
Flaxseeds	20%
Chia Seeds	14%
Sunflower Seeds	11%

Not everyone has the same proclivity, or liking, for foods, or the same nutritional requirements. But the body requires similar things for health and wellness, and we are all very much alike in numerous ways, having the same basic needs, the same general physiology, the same susceptibility to biological disharmony, the same susceptibility to many illnesses, and we share many of the same stresses, worries and fears that can influence our state of health. Nutritionists, whose voices have not been heard as much as those of ordinary diet proponents, have been telling us for years that ill-health and diseases of all types spring most often from one common source, namely, poor dietary practices.

The best diet is one that meets the energy and nutrient needs of the body and produces the least negative effects, such as toxicity, acidity and constipation. For most people, it means a diet consisting of a large volume of fresh, raw fruits and vegetables to meet the body's nutrient needs, and enough concentrated foods, such as nuts and seeds, to meet the body's energy needs.

"If you diligently heed the voice of the Lord your God and do what is right in His sight, give ear to His commandments and keep all His statutes, I will put none of the diseases on you which I have brought on the Egyptians." - Ex. 15:26.

The Importance of Apple Cider Vinegar and Honey

Apple cider vinegar (not the white distilled or wine vinegars) is known to assist in the digestion of foods. As explained in Victoria Boutenko's book, *Green for Life*, hydrochloric acid production in the stomach decreases after age 40. A low stomach acid condition is blamed for various nutritional deficiencies due to the inability of the body to adequately digest foods and absorb nutrients. It is also blamed for the greying of hair. Nutritional experts claim that supplementing the diet with apple cider vinegar helps to restore stomach acid to its proper levels.

Dr. N.W. Walker in his book Fresh Vegetable and Fruit Juices, states that apple cider vinegar contains malic acid, which is absent in white distilled and wine vinegars. Malic acid is beneficial to the body. All vinegars, including apple cider vinegar, are acidic, but as explained in his book, diluted apple cider vinegar is alkalizing to the body. In addition, malic acid can be stored in the body as glycogen for future use, and is known to promote healthy blood vessels, veins and arteries, and aid in coagulating the blood in establishing a normal menstrual flow.

Apple cider vinegar is made by fermenting crushed apples, which makes it different from other vinegars such as white or wine vinegars which are made by fermenting alcohol. Apple cider vinegar has the highest pH of any vinegar, 3.3 to 3.5. Other vinegars have a pH of around 2.4 making then more acidic. The lower the pH, the more acidic is the solution (pH is a logarithmic scale).

Raw, unpasteurized apple cider vinegar contains the "mother", which is a murky substance found at the bottom of the bottle. The mother is rich in enzymes, pectin (the soluble fiber found naturally in apples), and minerals including magnesium, phosphorus, calcium and potassium. There is some evidence that the malic acid in apple cider vinegar helps to release iron from foods so that it can be better utilized by the body, and that the high potassium content of ACV helps to restore mineral balance to the body.

One of the benefits of apple cider vinegar and honey is that it promotes sounder sleeps. Just a few teaspoons of apple cider vinegar and honey in a glass of water taken in the late afternoon or early evening can produce sounder sleep for the night.

Some incredible cures have been attributed to apple cider vinegar. An example is arthritis. For a complete discussion of how this long-practiced Vermont folklore cure has been used to cure arthritis, see the book, *The Cure for Arthritis*, or the books by Dr. D. C. Jarvis and Paul C. and Patricia Bragg that are listed in the Bibliography.

The following are recommended for the diet: 1) organic, raw, unpasteurized apple cider vinegar with the mother, and 2) organic, raw, unfiltered honey. Both are sold at whole food stores and on the Web.

Summary

While many fad diets claim to be the best yet for health, there is one way of eating that guarantees long-lasting health benefits, and that is the raw vegan diet. It is a complete shift in eating habits away from lifeless, cooked foods to living plant foods, the only foods that have life force properties that God and Nature intended for us to receive, which support all bodily functions and have the nutrients and enzymes the body needs to heal itself and sustain itself in health. If we follow God and do what He has asked of us, it will only lead to our happiness and eternal glory.

GMO Crops

Currently, according to the Web, there are ten (10) genetically modified food crops commercially available. They are listed below with the year they became commercially available. Other crops have been genetically modified as well, but they are either no longer commercially available because they were withdrawn from the market due to unfavorable reception, or they are in the process of being patented.

Soybeans, 1995

Squash, 1995

Corn (field and sweet), 1996

Cotton, 1996

Papaya, 1997

Canola (rapeseed), 1999

Alfalfa, 2006

Sugar beets, 2006

Potatoes, 2016

Apples, 2017

All the above foods are for human consumption (cottonseed oil is often used in food products), and some are also used for livestock feed.

Upwards of 75% of the refined and processed foods on supermarket shelves contain GMO products. GMO sweet corn and sugar beets are widely used in refined and processed foods as "sugar" or high-fructose corn syrup (HFCS). GMO soybeans are widely used as soy in many refined and processed foods. Soy is found in almost all baked goods and imitation dairy products, and also in alternative meat products such as veggie burgers. Soy derivatives include hydrolyzed plant protein (HPP), hydrolyzed soy protein (HSP) and/or hydrolyzed vegetable protein (HVP), which are added to a wide range of refined and processed foods, including soda, chips, salad dressings and soups.

GMO (Genetically Modified Organism) refers to a plant or animal (e.g., a fish) that is artificially created by inserting genes from one species into the DNA of another species. GE (Genetically Engineered) is another term used for genetically-altered foods.

Many GMO creations have been, and are now being, patented and released into our environment and food supply, and there seems to be no end in sight. Of course, if we buy all our foods "organic", that is, having the proper "Organic" label on them, then we should not have to worry about GMO foods, at least not for the present. This was covered in the last chapter under the section, "The Importance of Organic Foods."

One of the reasons for developing GMO crops was to make them more pesticide- and herbicide-resistant so they could tolerate lethal herbicides and pesticides that non-GMO crops cannot tolerate.

There are two main health concerns associated with consuming GMO crops. First, the highly poisonous pesticides and herbicides that are used on these crops may leave high residues on the crops or seep into the crops themselves. We know that the pesticides and herbicides used on non-GMO crops leave residues and can seep into the crops. See Appendix II.

The second danger is the risk to human health of the Bt (Bacillus thuringiensis) toxin, which is genetically inserted into the DNA of the crop species. The cells of the species that are modified are genetically engineered to include the Bt toxin in order to kill the pests that feed on the crops. The toxin acts as a delayed-action bomb that goes off when pests eat the crops. Crops that have been modified to take the Bt toxin include corn, cotton, and soybeans.

The flurry of reports that were the rage of the 1990s and early 2000s about the health hazards of GMO foods are no longer in the news. The reports have become much less frequent, replaced by carefully-worded reports and articles that are sponsored by food industry advocates of the food industry, that support the continued use of GMO crops. The principal pro-GMO argument is that GMO crops resist many food viruses and pests, thus making them more available to more people. However, these reports and articles, many of which are on the Web, fail to adequately address, for many people, the earlier-identified dangers of consuming these foods. As a result of these developments, public attention as a whole has shifted away from the dangers of GMOs to other concerns.

There is a scarcity of scientific studies on humans to justify the health risks that are associated with the above-described dangers. But there have been numerous reports showing that human health is adversely affected by these crops. These reports are not limited to the adverse health effects on farm workers who spray the pesticides and herbicides on the crops, but include people who eat the GMO crops.

One of the difficulties in assessing studies done on the human health effects of GMO crops is the fact the evaluation of GE herbicide-resistant crops is conducted by USDA, their evaluation when the crops can be consumed by people is conducted by FDA, while the herbicides are assessed by EPA when there are new potential exposures.[9]

However, it stands to reason that if the strong pesticides and herbicides that are sprayed on GMO crops adversely affect the health of GMO farm workers, then the same poisons may adversely affect the health of people who consume the GMO crops. And, if eating GMO crops that have the Bt toxin kills insects, then eating the crops may adversely affect human health in some way.

At the time of this writing, there are no requirements to label GMO food "GMO" or "GE" or anything else to alert consumers of what they are buying. This is despite opinion polls that show that up to 90 percent of Americans want GMO foods labeled.

"Is there any intelligent being who is so naïve as to assume that the poisons will be less devastating to the human body, with its endlessly more intricate and delicate living mechanism?" - Dr. Lars-Eric Essen.

On the raw vegan diet, only raw, natural foods are consumed. Therefore, if you are on the diet you should not worry about consuming GMO foods, unless you buy non-organic produce. In that case, you should ensure that the produce is not a GMO food by checking the list above or an updated list as time goes by. If any of the foods you buy are purchased non-organic, that is, not

---

[9] 2016 NCBI report on the Web entitled, "Human Health Effects of Genetically Engineered Crops."

having a "USDA Organic" "CCOF Organic" or OTCO label on them (as discussed previously), then they are likely to be GMO foods.

Not all varieties of foods that are listed above have been genetically modified, at least not as yet. For example, there are over a hundred varieties of apples, one of my favorite foods, but only one variety, Artic apples, has been genetically modified as of this writing according to the Web.

Potatoes that are genetically modified include the White Russet potatoes which are used worldwide in fast-food restaurants for fries.

"The huge jump in childhood food allergies in the US is in the news often, but most reports fail to consider a link to a recent radical change in America's diet. Beginning in 1996, bacteria, virus and other genes have been artificially inserted to the DNA of soy, corn, cottonseed and canola plants. These unlabeled genetically modified (GM) foods carry a risk of triggering life-threatening allergic reactions, and evidence collected over the past decade now suggests that they are contributing to higher allergy rates." - Jeffery M. Smith, from a Web article.

It would seem that the wide-spread consumption of GMO crops in our society is the population study, or test, that these crops will have to see what happens to human health as a result of eating them. It also appears that everyone who consumes GMO crops is an individual test case. It appears that we are all guinea pigs in a gigantic experiment, and no one knows for sure what the outcome will be. That is not a good way to conduct a scientific study on human heath, nor is it good policy!

In addition to the human health dangers, GMO crops contaminate non-GE counterparts, for example corn. Cross-pollination has led to the widespread contamination of non-GMO corn crops. Controlling the spread of GE contamination has proven to be all but impossible. Since this threat is so real and prevalent, it is best to restrict one's diet to food types that have not been genetically engineered.

Two popular DVDs have explored and documented the dangers of GMO crops, *Genetic Roulette* and *The GMO Trilogy*. Both are by Jeffery M. Smith, who authored the books *Seeds of Deception* and *Genetic Roulette* that the movies are based on.

Although the controversy about the health hazards of eating GMO crops seems to have faded into the past, we need to keep vigilant on what is going on in the food industry if we wish to improve and maintain our health, especially since so much health information today is being controlled by vested interests that care much more about their profit than our health.

The Dangers of Cooked Foods

"If you eat living food, the same will quicken you, but if you kill your food the dead food will kill you also. For life comes only from life, and from death always comes death." - Attributed to Jesus, *The Essene Gospel of Peace, Book One.*

Nutritional experts have stressed for years that cooked foods are harmful to human health, and that the cooking of foods done at home and in restaurants, and in the food factories that manufacture canned, bottled and jarred foods, reduces the food value of the foods by altering their chemical properties and destroying important food constituents such as enzymes and nutrients, which also includes vitamins. They have also been telling us that cooked foods of almost any kind create acidity in the body. It is now known that cooking and the refining and processing of foods are responsible for the development of many of the sicknesses and diseases that plague humankind.

As stated previously, Americans eat more cooked food than any people on earth, and spend more money on doctor bills and healthcare than any people on earth. The fast food franchises, as well as other eating establishments, grill, fry, bake, and steam-heat their foods, or use dehydrated foods that have already been refined and processed using these methods. It has been known for years that these methods destroy important food components such as enzymes, vitamins and other nutrients, and also alter the chemical properties of the foods.

Robert Morse in his book, *The Detox Miracle Sourcebook*, explains how cooking dramatically decreases the molecular energy of foods, since heat affects the electrons of the food molecules and alters their molecular structure. However, when we eat raw foods, their high electromagnetic energy is transferred to the body and its cells.

Dr. N. W. Walker in many of his books, such as *Colon Health* and *Become Younger*, tells us that foods are demagnetized when they are cooked, and that only living (raw, uncooked) plant foods have the magnetic properties that are needed by the body. He states that the fiber we consume in our diets should be comprised of the fiber or roughage of raw plant foods, and that if this fiber comes from cooked foods, it will be demagnetized, or devitalized, to the extent that it will pass through the system with little or no benefit.

In addition, cooked, starchy foods leave a plaster-like coating on the walls of the large intestine (colon). This coating builds up over time as more of these foods are consumed, which decreases the capacity to absorb vital nutrients and prevents food from being completely digested. More is provided about this in the next chapter.

Cooked food is any food heated above 118° F. It includes almost every kind of food that comes in an airtight sealed package (bag, box, can, jar, bottle, etc.). For comparison purposes, a hot shower is 105° F, typical pasteurization temperature is 160° F, water boils at 212° F, canned foods are heated during the canning process to 240-250° F, and microwave and stove ovens heat foods to 300-500° F.

"Cooked food is dead, and actually unsuitable as nourishment for the digestive processes of all animals, including human beings." - Dr. Ann Wigmore, *Be Your Own Doctor*.

Cooked foods (plant or animal) are foods devoid of life. They require additional energy from the body to be digested and assimilated, energy that could be used for other purposes, such as healing. Cooked foods contain coagulated and unusable proteins and dead enzymes that are toxic to the body.

According to Dr. D. C. Jarvis in his book, *Folk Medicine*, cooking reduces potassium 70% for carrots, onions, potatoes, pumpkin and spinach, 60% for cauliflower, cabbage, peas, asparagus, string beans and Brussel sprouts, and 50% for corn, beets and tomatoes. Potassium is needed for the proper functioning of the nervous system.

Cooked foods are tasteless compared to raw foods, which is why they require condiments, such as salt, pepper and sugar, and combinations of them. Many of the condiments have deleterious effects on the body, including refined sugar and refined salt, as explained in this book.

Because cooked foods are dead foods and deficient in nutrients, our hunger is not sated when we eat them in small portions, so we overeat. However, overeating is known to be a precursor of many health complications, including obesity and disease.

As stated previously, raw plant foods are foods as-found in nature. They are not cooked or chemically altered, and they do not contain preservatives, artificial colors or flavors. Raw plant foods are living foods with their natural life force properties intact. It is this life force that is imparted to us when we eat raw plant foods.

The dangers of cooked foods discussed so far are sufficient in themselves to justify eliminating all cooked foods from your diet. But cooking of foods has more dangers. If food is browned by heat treatment, such as by broiling, baking or deep frying, dangerous chemicals are created, such as advanced glycation end-products (AGEs), which have been linked to diabetes and heart disease. This was discussed in a previous chapter.

Furthermore, nutritional experts assert that cooked food is addictive. Like other addictions, the cooked food addiction gets stronger with continued use. Details are provided later in this book on how to kick this addiction.

The consensus of modern nutritional experts, including Norman W. Walker, Robert Morse, Arnold Ehret, Theresa Mitchell, Ann Wigmore, Edward Howell, David Wolfe, Herbert M. Shelton, O.L.M. Abramowski, Fred Hirsch, Harvey Diamond, Bernard Jensen, Professor Spira, Kristina Carrillo-Bucaram, Victoria Boutenko, Joe Alexander and Paavo Airola, is that the consumption of cooked foods is detrimental to human health, and that they should not be eaten.

Enzymes

Enzymes are life-force factors, biological catalysts that are necessary for life processes. They are substances that make life possible. Enzymes are needed for every chemical reaction that takes place in the body. It is claimed that no mineral, vitamin or hormone can do any work without enzymes. The body's ability to digest and assimilate foods is totally dependent on enzymes.

"I attest that the kitchen stove and its big brothers, the heat treatment machinery in food factories, are responsible for destroying a whole category of food elements, namely the heat-sensitive exogenous food enzymes." - Dr. Edward Howell, *Enzyme Nutrition*.

Raw plant foods are replete with enzymes as provided by nature to facilitate their digestion and assimilation in the body. According to Dr. Edward Howell, raw plant foods have all the enzymes needed for human consumption. The pancreas produces enzymes, but you'll always have exogenous enzymes if you eat raw, uncooked foods.

"To get enzymes from food, one must eat raw food. The heat used in cooking destroys all food enzymes and forces the organism to produce more enzymes, thus enlarging digestive organs, especially the pancreas." - Dr. Edward Howell, *Enzyme Nutrition.*

The nutritional experts believe that eating cooked food requires the body to use up its enzyme reserves for digestion and assimilation. More specifically, the enzymes of the body must perform the job of digesting cooked foods. This depletes the enzyme reserves of the body, making it increasingly difficult as time goes by to properly digest foods. As a result, we become weaker and more fatigued, despite the amount of food we consume. In addition, energy that is used by the body to digest cooked foods is diverted away from other badly needed bodily functions such as self-cleansing and healing.

One of the things that interests me in particular about the dangers of eating cooked foods is that Dr. Howell in his book, *Enzyme Nutrition,* states that enzyme activity in the body becomes weaker with age. He also states that based on clinical studies performed on animals and humans, each of us is given a limited supply of enzymes at birth, and that when the supply is depleted, we die, and the faster we use up our enzyme supply the shorter our life will be. This is one of the main reasons why we should avoid all cooked foods. It implies that the more cooked foods we eat, the sooner our life will come to an end.

Again, cooked foods are devoid of enzymes because heat destroys them. Furthermore, cooked foods cause us to look older than we really are. They make wrinkles appear, especially on the face.

Dr. Ann Wigmore, in her book, *Be Your Own Doctor*, states that when food is cooked it permits tumors and cancer growth to build, but when food is eaten raw the cancer and other growths immediately begin to shrink. This indicates that cooked foods are precursors of human disease.

Surprisingly, there is a dearth of information on the Web about the harmful effects of cooked foods on human health. Many of the websites queried for this information actually encourage eating cooked as part of a healthy diet. Again, books have the answers to many of the important questions about foods and nutrition.

Raw plant foods may be sliced, diced, run through a food processor, blender, etc., as long as they are not cooked. They can be eaten by themselves or combined with other raw foods if properly combined (see chapter on "Proper Food Combinations").

"Eating raw foods is the number one activity which preserves enzymes and maximizes health." - Gabriel Cousens, *Conscious Eating*.

The conclusion of this chapter is obvious. We should eat as many enzyme-rich foods as possible, which are raw plant foods, and avoid all cooked foods.

Vegetables that are so often cooked can be eaten raw. We can eat raw potatoes, as long as we don't eat green ones that can be toxic. Also, there are plenty of raw plant foods that satisfy cravings for cooked foods and sweets. For example, what is more satisfying than a ripe peach or mango? You can snack on pecans and honey, cacao nibs or bee pollen soaked in water, bananas with Mission figs or dates and sweet apples.

Substituting living plant foods for cooked foods solves all of the problems described in this chapter.

For more information about how cooked foods are harmful to human health, I refer you to the books listed in the Bibliography by Norman W. Walker, Robert Morse, Arnold Ehret, Theresa Mitchell, Ann Wigmore, Edward Howell, David Wolfe, Herbert M. Shelton, O.L.M. Abramowski, Fred Hirsch, Harvey Diamond, Bernard Jensen, Professor Spira, Kristina Carrillo-Bucaram, Victoria Boutenko, Joe Alexander and Paavo Airola.

The dangers of eating cooked foods may shock or surprise many people because most of us grew up eating cooked foods and have learned to like them. Hopefully, this chapter will serve as a re-thinking starting point about how cooked foods should be viewed.

The Dangers of Starchy Foods

Many of the contributors to our understanding of the causes of human diseases were famous nutritionists, including Professor Arnold Ehret, who was popular in Germany in the early 1900s, and later in America.

Ehret was probably the first scientist to recognize that mucus-forming foods cause waste obstruction in the body, and that the obstruction causes disease. In his book, *The Cause and Cure of Human Illness,* he states that there are two main reasons for human disease: 1) constipation caused by mucus-producing foods, and 2) overeating, i.e., eating more than is necessary, more than the system can handle, more than it actually needs.

In his landmark book, *The Mucusless Diet Healing System*, first published in 1922, Ehret released to the world his incredible findings about how optimum health can be achieved by eating a starch-free diet consisting of fresh raw fruits, leafy greens and non-starchy vegetables (mucusless foods) which he claimed was the optimal diet for human health. These are the natural foods of man (Genesis' "fruits and herbs"). The book is considered by many nutritional experts to be the definitive work on the prevention and curing of human disease through diet and fasting.

Some of the dangers of eating starchy foods have been discussed in the chapter on "The Causes of Disease." As mentioned in that chapter, Ehret healed himself of Bright's disease (a kidney disease), and cured many hopeless cases of chronic diseases by putting his patients on his mucusless diet and fasting regimen. Many of the patients were very serious cases with terminal diseases, and lay on their deathbeds. Many had gone through other therapies and followed the advice given, including strict diets, but without success. He also cured those who suffered from degenerative diseases, both acute and chronic. After following his mucusless diet for only a short time, all of his patients regained their health.

Starchy foods include wheat, corn, rice, white and red potatoes, beans of all kinds and peas. They also include food products made from these foods, such as bread, pasta, cereals, pastries, corn starch, etc. (Note that carrots and beets are non-starchy foods as discussed in the chapter on "Proper Food Combinations.")

Many nutritional experts concur that starchy foods cause disease in the human body. The reason is that they cause paste-like plaque to coat, or plate-out, on the insides of the large intestine, or colon, which hinders the absorption of nutrients in the body. They believe that people are nutrient deficient and constipated because of the large amounts of starchy foods they habitually eat.

The clogging up process resulting from the consumption of starchy foods can be easily proven on the raw vegan diet by simply eating white flour products, such as pizza or while flour bread, for several days. The result is constipation and difficult bowel movements, whereas stopping the consumption of these foods results in the return of regular and smooth defecations.

The clogging up of the intestines caused by starchy foods causes intestinal bacteria to multiply inordinately which releases poisons into the blood stream. The state of constipation is the primary cause of illness and disease in the human body according to Dr. N. W. Walker, Professor Arnold Ehret, Dr. Ann Wigmore, Fred Hirsch, Karyn Calabrese, Professor Spira, and other nutritionists.

The degree of being constipated correlates with the number of meals eaten per day versus the number of defecations per day. In other words, if a person is not having as many bowel movements per day as meals taken per day, they are constipated, and the lower the ratio the more constipated they are.

Dr. N. W. Walker found that the plaster-like coating formed by starchy foods builds up and increases in thickness over time until only a small opening remains in the large intestine for food residue to pass out of the system. This conclusion is based on Walker's examination of thousands of X-rays of the colons of chronically ill patients. He believed that starchy foods were primarily responsible for this obstruction of the colon and the resulting spread of poisons throughout the body.

Walker believed that any treatment of disease would be totally ineffective unless the accumulated starchy plaque that has formed in the large intestine over the years has been washed out of the colon by colonic irrigations. This conclusion is based on his healing of chronically ill patients by having them undergo a series of colonics. It was the cleansing action of the colonics that caused the plaque to be released from the walls of the colon, and when that occurred the health of his patients was restored. This is exactly what Arnold Ehret and others have stressed in their books.

Most people are not aware of the dangers of starchy foods, as they are not aware of the dangers of cooked foods. At the time of this writing, I could not find any websites that discussed the harmful effects that starches have on the large intestine (colon), or that attribute starchy foods as a cause of human disease.

"If you consumed a lifetime supply of dairy, meat and other mucus-producing foods, you may have built up many layers of glue-like toxins on your colon walls. Although some waste can pass through your intestines daily, leading you to believe that your body is adequately digesting the food you eat, the lining of your intestines will continue to toughen and narrow." - Karyn Calabrese, *Soak Your Nuts*.

"No system of healing can be permanently effective until the eliminative organs have been thoroughly cleansed of accumulated waste matter and at the same time all grain and starchy foods have been eliminated from one's diet." - Norman W. Walker, *Become Younger*.

Let me ask you a simple question. Are you sure you want to eat that next slice of bread or bowl of rice?

The Dangers of Refined Sugar

Refined sugar includes white sugar (aka table sugar), brown sugar, high-fructose corn syrup (HFCS), maltose, dextrose, and artificial sweeteners such as saccharin, acesulfame, aspartame, neotame, and sucralose. These substances are produced using intensive heat. As such, their enzymes are destroyed. They have zero fiber, and there is nothing of nutritional value in them. Refined sugar is often referred to as empty calorie food. But refined sugar cannot really be classed as food since it does not contain any vitamins or minerals. As seen in this chapter, refined sugar is a threat to human health.

It is said that the sweetening of foods has become a necessity in order to make foods more palatable, meaning that they would not taste well to the majority of people if they were not sweetened. But think about this for a moment. Having become accustomed to eating foods sweetened with refined sugar, many of us can no longer enjoy foods unless they are sweetened.

The increased use of refined sugar in our culture is responsible not only for desensitizing our taste buds to the point where many of us can no longer appreciate natural tastes and flavors, but their use the use in foods and drinks is a serious health problem. We have lost a great deal in the industrialization of foods and drinks. The way things are going, the continued use of refined sugar does not portend well for the future of our society.

There is overwhelming evidence that unnatural forms of sugar are destructive to the human organism. Refined sugar has a detrimental effect on tooth enamel, causing dental caries. It causes diabetes and destroys the gastrointestinal tract and alimentary canal. According to the Web, refined sugar detrimentally affects the health of 60–90% of schoolchildren and almost all adults in this country. It causes cancer, vision disorders and pyorrhea (shrinkage of gums and loosening of teeth), as well as other health disorders. According to Dr. Norman W. Walker, when we eat or drink anything that contains refined sugar, the pancreas is overworked, which causes its inflammation and results in pancreatitis.

According to USDA, people who consume a lot of sugar (as most people do) have the lowest intakes of essential nutrients, including calcium and vitamins A, C, and B-12. It is of particular danger to children and teens who need the most nutrients but consume the most sugar.

The commercial reason for the large-scale sweetening of foods and drinks in this country was discussed in the chapter on "The Foods We Should Eat and Why." The food industry has for years designed food products to titillate the taste buds and activate the reward centers of the brain, seeing the result of it in the sales of the foods and drinks in which the products are added.

The only sugars that are of any value to human health are the natural sugars found in raw fruits and vegetables and in unrefined bee products such as honey and bee pollen.

When we eat raw fruits and vegetables, we receive the natural sugars that are in them, plus the fiber, and they are well utilized by the body. We also receive rich amounts of antioxidants and phytochemicals, which, along with the fiber, curb the rapid assimilation of sugar in the bloodstream and block its negative effects.

We can satisfy our sweet tooth by eating sweet fruits. If you've never tried sugar-free dried mango or natural Turkish figs together with bananas, you will be very pleasantly surprised when you do.

As discussed in the chapter on "GMO Crops," GMO sweet corn and sugar beets are widely used in refined and processed foods, as well as condiments, as "sugar" or "high-fructose corn syrup (HFCS)."

For health, we should strictly avoid foods that contain refined sugar, and make fruits, vegetables and bee products our choices for snacks and for fighting the blues.

Abiding by Nature's Laws

Natural laws govern our world. They include the laws of physics that encompass the mysterious forces of electromagnetism, gravity and the nuclear forces, and also the laws of biological processes, including life itself. Natural laws are always in effect, and they apply to everyone in every generation.

All creatures seem to be perfectly attuned and adjusted to these laws, except for man. We are constantly challenging or testing Nature in one way or another. Our free will, which other creatures do not have, and which sets us apart from the other creatures perhaps more than anything else, enables us to question the validity of natural laws. But Nature has a way of punishing and even eliminating people who break her laws.

In the province of Nature, things happen to us as a consequence of the way that we choose to live, the choices that we make in life, including our food choices and eating habits. For example, if I combine my foods improperly, I can expect to get a stomachache or headache. If I eat the Standard American Diet, I can expect to be the recipient of a large number of food-related health disorders that are linked to meat and dairy products and to devitalized, refined and processed foods.

The law of cause and effect is one of Nature's laws. It happens to be the foundation of the scientific method, which is the basis for all the discoveries and inventions made in the sciences, including chemistry, physics, geology, biology and the medical sciences. The law of cause and effect is observed in many clinical trials and studies that are conducted on human health and nutrition each year that show a direct relationship between the diseases of humankind and diet. Some of these trials and studies are documented in articles of the scientific and medical professions, many of which are available on the Internet, and some are cited in this book as well as in the books that are listed in the Bibliography.

If you don't want the effect, do something about the causes.

"The present ignorance of the laws underlying normal health is now, in this century, the greatest of all the past centuries, and is evidenced by the deterioration of the so-called civilized people health-wise." - Arnold Ehret, *Physical Fitness Through a Superior Diet, Fasting, and Dietetics.*

As discussed in previous chapters, many medical researchers and nutritionists claim that the cause of many human diseases are the foods that are commonly consumed, rather than normal processes of aging, such as natural "wear and tear" of the body. It is my belief that this claim will be proven to everyone's satisfaction in the years to come, impacting many popular beliefs regarding age-related health issues. An example is the degenerative disease of arthritis. Many nutritionists, including Dr. Ann Wigmore, believe that arthritis is caused by harmful dietary practices.

Raw plant foods have their enzymes intact to assist the body in their digestion, but cooking destroys food enzymes. The lack of enzymes in cooked foods causes the body to draw on its enzyme reserves for their digestion. Many nutritionists, such as Dr. Edward Howell, contend that this is one of the causes of degeneration in the body.

"Among the many thousands of species of creatures living on the earth, only humans and some of their domesticated animals (dogs, cats) try to live without food enzymes. And only these transgressors of nature's laws are penalized with defective health." - Dr. Edward Howell, *Enzyme Nutrition.*

Fasting (simply eating less) is one of Nature's powerful ways of cleansing the body of the harmful effects of improper diet and too much eating. When animals get sick, they instinctively abstain from food. But man seems to have lost this instinct, if he ever had it.

It is our duty to understand Nature's laws if we wish to live a healthy life, one that is free of health disorders, including diseases. The appreciation of the power of a natural law at work in us is one of the most profound things that we can ever experience.

Eating foods with their enzymes intact, undestroyed by heat (raw plant foods), avoiding the dangers of cooked and starchy foods, practicing proper food combinations, and curing health issues through a combination of proper diet and fasting are only a few examples of dietary practices that adhere to the laws of Nature. You will learn about these things, and more, in this book.

God lets us make our own choices. He does not prevent us from ruining our health. He permits us to exercise the free will that He has given us to make our own decisions. We have to face the consequences of our actions.

Another law of nature is the need for adequate rest. In our fast-paced society, with its unrelenting demands on our time and money, our minds cry out for adequate rest. We are told that eight hours of sleep per night are required for health, but many of us get less than five. Is this abiding by Nature's laws?

The body always lets us know how we are treating it. Under-standing and heeding the warning signals the body provides helps us to maintain ourselves in concert with the laws of nature. As mentioned previously, the body can take a lot of abuse before it starts to show the ill effects of deterioration. But when that occurs, a person could be, health-wise speaking, at the point of no return. By staying proactive in this regard, we can avoid many of the health disorders, including diseases, that stalk our society.

This reveals a basic truth about our lives. The consequences of our choices are different than their effects. To avoid the perils of constipation, one must not eat foods that cause it, notwithstanding the joy one may have in doing so.

We must be concerned about the foods, the water and the air that we take into our bodies, and with the sleep and other forms of rest that we get, because they affect our chemistry and physiology for good or for bad. Moreover, we must accept Nature's laws and stop trying to alter them to meet our own desires.

"Healing is no accident. All nature heals itself when causes are removed and the conditions of health supplied." - Dr. Herbert M. Shelton.

"It must always be understood that one has to strive to go forward in the service of our Lord and in self-knowledge." - St. Teresa of Avila.

Proper Food Combinations

"Cook not, neither mix all things one with another, lest your bowels become as steaming bogs...for I tell you truly, if you mix together all sorts of food in your body, then the peace of your body will cease, and endless war will rage in you." - Attributed to Jesus, *The Essene Gospel of Peace, Book One.*

Before food can nourish the body, it must be digested. Digestion is a chemical process that breaks down food into constituents that can be assimilated by the body. Digestion starts in the mouth with saliva and continues in the stomach where digestive juices, or gastric juices, are secreted to break down the food. The job of digestion is not finished until the food travels through the small and large intestines and the wastes pass out of the body.

Food combination laws are rules of nature that are based on the principle that different types of foods require different times for digestion, and cause the secretion in the stomach of different types of gastric juices, some being more acidic, some less acidic. If we eat foods that cause more alkaline (less acidic) gastric juices for their digestion together with foods that require more acidic juices for their digestion, the juices combine, resulting in food in the stomach that is difficult to digest. This leads to a variety of complications, such as stomachaches, headaches and fermentation, and, when the food passes through the intestines, putrefaction, gas and the breeding of parasites.

When foods are difficult to digest, the energy reserves of the body are called into play to assist in the job of digestion. It should not be surprising that you feel tired after eating a big meal of improperly combined foods -- the traditional nap after a Thanksgiving dinner.

The stomach does not decide what foods to put in it. It leaves that job to the brain.

The Web adequately covers many aspects of proper food combining. A good website on proper food combining at the time of this writing is: https: //www.acidalkalinediet.net/correct-food-combining-principles.php.

However, some Web articles on food combining do not stand up to careful scrutiny. For example, some tell us that combining nuts with sweet fruits is an improper food combination. But based on my experience, and what nutritional experts tell us, fatty nuts (like walnuts and pecans) combine well with some sweet fruits, such as bananas and dates. Other sweet fruits, such as apples; that have a high water content, can make the nuts indigestible.

In *The Sunfood Diet Success System*, David Wolfe explains that nuts are actually fat-dominant, not protein-dominant, foods because they consist mostly of fat (see the table provided in the Nuts and Seeds section of this book). He explains that the fat in nuts and seeds allows the natural sugar in sweet fruit to be time-released, which helps digestion and provides more long-term energy. Combining sweet fruits with fatty nuts and seeds is an acceptable food combination, contrary to some of the articles on the Web.

The food combination laws should be learned, even if one or two of them are not correctly stated on the Web. The laws that are not correctly stated on the Web at least err on the safe side so that by observing them you will not be hurting yourself. Set goals for yourself to rigidly put the laws into practice.

The rules of food combining are soundly rooted in physiology and thoroughly tested by experience.

"More than sixty years spent in feeding the well and the sick, the weak and the strong, the old and the young, have demonstrated that a change to correctly combined meals is followed by an immediate improvement in health as a consequence of lightening the load the digestive organs have to carry, thus assuring better digestion." - Herbert M. Shelton, *Food Combining Made Easy*.

I enjoy many foods by themselves, but I'm an inveterate mixer. I prefer to mix my foods, to combine them. I learned the food combination laws the hard way, by trial and error, and suffered all the resulting stomachaches of improperly combined foods. Very probably, you will learn them the hard way too. It took me about a year to put the laws into practice without making further mistakes.

Five of the food combination laws that are important on any diet, including the raw vegan diet, are as follows.

1. Don't Eat Proteins with Starches

Example: Spirulina or hemp seed (both protein foods) eaten with Maca (a starchy food).

2. Don't Eat Starches with Acid Fruit

Example: Potatoes or peas (both starchy foods) eaten with tomatoes (acid fruit).

Note that tomatoes combine well with leafy greens and fatty plant foods like avocados.

3. Don't Eat Starches with Sweet or Sub-Acid Fruit

Example: Beans or peas (starchy foods) added to green smoothies that contain sweet or sub-acid fruit.

I have my own rule for this – don't add vegetables other than leafy greens to green smoothies. I've had too many stomachaches from breaking this law, so I make it easier to remember by excluding all vegetables (except greens) from my green smoothies which contain sweet fruit.

4. Don't Eat Sweet Fruit with Acid Fruit

Example: Pineapple (an acid fruit) eaten with bananas or dates (sweet fruit).

Note that sweet fruit combines well with sub-acid fruits, such as apricots.

5. Don't Eat Proteins with Sweet Fruit

Example: Hemp seed with dates. Hemp seed is 30% protein. Higher protein foods, such as spirulina, are even worse combinations with sweet fruit because they cause severe gas resulting from the fermentation that occurs. Bananas are an exception because they combine well with nuts and seeds.

The above food combination laws cover some of the errors typically made on the raw vegan diet. Additional food combination laws should also be learned. As explained previously, you can learn about them on the Web.

Greens (green leafy vegetables) are the only foods that combine well with all other foods, including other greens.

To aid in preparing meals, the digestion times required for different types of foods should also be learned. Obviously, we should not combine foods that require completely different digestion times. Digestion times for different foods are adequately covered on the Web. Typically, digestion times and proper food combinations go hand in hand.

When the food combination laws are obeyed, digestion is greatly improved and overall well-being is enhanced. When food combination laws are broken, stomachaches, headaches, excessive flatulence, or other complications can and do result, which can quickly turn what started out to be a good day into a bad one.

"Improved digestion results in general improvement in all the functions of life. Many and great are the benefits to flow from improved digestion." - Dr. Herbert M. Shelton, Food Combining Made Easy.

How to Determine the Starch Content of Foods

Food labels (Nutrition Facts Labels) typically give the amount of total carbohydrates, sugar and fiber, but not the amount of starch in the food. The starch content might be published on the Web, but if it's not, here's how to determine the starch content of any food from its Nutrition Facts Label.

From the food label on the product package, or as given on the Web, get the weights in grams of total carbohydrates, sugars and fiber and plug them into the following equation:

Starch = Carbs – (Sugars + Fiber).

Example 1: Maca. On the Web, the Nutrition Facts Label for Maca lists, for a 100g serving: 71g carbs, 32g sugars and 7g fiber.

Starch (g) = 71g – (32g + 7g) = 71g – 39g = 32g

32g/100g = 32%

Maca is 32% starch. Since starch content is a considerable portion of Maca, it is a starchy vegetable.

Example 2: Carrots. Per the Web, a 61g serving of carrots has 6g carbs, 2.9g sugars and 1.7g fiber.

Starch (g) = 6g – (2.9g + 1.7g) = 6g – 4.8g = 1.2g

1.2g/61g = 2%

Carrots are 2% starch. Since the starch content of carrots is very low, it is a non-starchy vegetable.

Many articles on the Web differ on whether carrots are starchy or non-starchy vegetables. Some articles say carrots are starchy vegetables while others say they are non-starchy vegetables. This is another example of conflicting information found on the Web.

Example 3: Beets. Per the Web, a 100g serving of beets has 10g carbs, 7g sugars and 2.8g fiber.

Similar to the above computations, beets are 0.2% starch. It is a non-starchy vegetable.

Example 4: Turnips. Per the Web, a 122g serving of turnips has 8g carbs, 4.6g sugars and 2.2g fiber.

Similar to the above computations, turnips are 0.1% starch. It is a non-starchy vegetable.

Example 5: Cinnamon. Per the Web, a 7.8g serving of cinnamon has: 6g carbs, 4.1g sugars and 0.2g fiber.

Similar to the above computations, cinnamon is 21% starch. Cinnamon is a starchy food. It should not be used with protein foods or with sweet or sub-acid fruit.

As the proper combination of hydrocarbons in your vehicle's fuel determines how it runs, so your life will run smoothly if your foods are eaten in their proper combinations. In my opinion, if positive feedback is not received by the body on any food that is eaten, no matter what the type or variety -- fruit, vegetable, Superfood, herb or any other kind of food -- then that food should either be eaten in a more ripe condition, in smaller quantities, in proper combinations with other foods, or it should be avoided. The body is no fool. It recognizes foods that disagree with it or do it harm by giving us warning signals. Our job then is to correctly interpret these signals.

The Blood

"The life of the flesh is in the blood." - Lev. 17:11.

This chapter describes the effects that foods have on blood health and shows how to interpret your own blood condition.

Blood is life. As the poets claim, it is the song of the lark, the blush on the cheek, the spring of the lamb. It is the sacred wine in the silver chalice. Down through the ages, blood has been the price men paid for freedom, and so it is today. Blood is our most preciously guarded possession.

Nutritionists tell us that the quality of the blood starts changing within a few hours after eating a meal. Blood cells, like other cells of the body, are continually being replaced. Old cells are being replaced by new cells. The new cells are constructed from the raw materials that foods and drinks provide. The quality of the blood depends a great deal on the quality of the foods that are eaten. When we eat cooked foods, including refined and processed foods, blood cells are constructed of inferior-quality building materials, materials that are devoid of the life force properties that raw plant foods possess.

"Dead atoms and dead molecules cannot rejuvenate or re-generate the cells of the body. Such food results in cell starvation and this in turn causes sickness and disease." - Norman W. Walker, *Water Can Undermine Your Health*.

As discussed in the chapter on "The Causes of Disease," acidity is a blood condition mainly brought on by eating too many acid-producing foods. When we eat foods typical of a cooked meat and/or pasteurized milk diet, which are acidic foods, the blood becomes thick and heavy which causes clogging in the tissues and is known to adversely affect the arteries and lymphatic system, and cause poor circulation and elevated blood pressure. When we eat whole plant foods such as raw fruits, vegetables and leafy greens, the blood's condition becomes normal, which is alkaline, and is not thickened which results in improved circulation and reduced blood pressure.

"Animal foods cannot build good blood; in fact, do not build human blood at all, because of the biological fact that man is by nature a fruit eater. Look at the juice of a ripe blackberry, black cherry or black grapes. Doesn't it almost resemble your blood? Can any reasonable man prove that half-decayed "muscle tissue" builds better blood?" - Arnold Ehret, *Mucusless Diet Healing System*.

Berg's Tables, provided in Appendix I, list common foods that are "acid-forming" or "acid-binding". According to the tables, meat and grain products are the most acid-forming foods, whereas fruits and vegetables are the most acid-binding foods.

Almost all raw plant foods are alkaline, or become alkaline in the body. Fruits of the Citrus genus (oranges, grapefruit, etc.) are alkalizing in the body despite their initial acidity. If we ate nothing but raw fruits, leafy greens and vegetables, our blood chemistry would be alkaline most of the time. The times when it would not be so would be in times of stress, or when we are exposed to environmental toxins, or are taking alcohol, caffeine or medication. Grains, most legumes, and most commonly eaten nuts are acid-forming (and mucus-forming) foods to some extent.

The chlorophyll in leafy green vegetables cleanses and alkalizes the blood. The body converts chlorophyll into heme, an iron compound that is part of hemoglobin, to produce red blood cells. Unfortunately, many Americans do not eat greens except in small amounts, such as lettuce in fast food sandwiches, which is one of the reasons why many people in this country are lacking in vitamins, antioxidants, and the therapeutic properties that plant foods have. Greens include spinach, kale, chard, lettuces, cabbages, collard greens and mustard greens. The importance of eating greens for health is discussed throughout this book.

As discussed in the chapter on "The Causes of Disease," homeostasis is the tendency of the body to maintain itself in stable chemical equilibrium. Health is said to be a balancing act with the body trying to balance or stabilize itself to a normal or alkaline blood condition. Obviously, the effectiveness at doing this is encumbered or enhanced by the foods that are eaten, and how they are eaten. An acidic blood condition is typically caused by a nutrient deficient diet. If the diet is continued, the blood condition worsens to where the body's attempts at homeostasis are not sufficient in neutralizing the acidic condition. The acids the body cannot neutralize and expel as waste get stored in the tissues and joints of the body which can lead to diseases.

Two examples of the effects of a poor blood condition are anemia, a condition of not having enough healthy red blood cells, and deep-vein thrombosis, which is blood clotting. Healthy blood does not produce these disorders.

According to Dr. Michael Greger's book, *How Not To Die*, plant-based diets have been shown to reduce the risk of blood cancers by 50%.

pH Balance

Nature's way is for the human body to maintain its blood in an alkaline pH range of 7.35 - 7.45, the range that the body tries to maintain at all times through the process of homeostasis. pH is a term used in chemistry for the amount of acidity or alkalinity of an aqueous solution. The pH scale runs from 0 to 14, with a pH of 7 being neutral, a pH of less than 7 being acidic, and a pH greater than 7 being alkaline.

The basal pH of gastric juices secreted by the glands of the stomach is strongly acidic, with a range of 1.5 - 3.5. The pH in the stomach changes when food is in the stomach, and is influenced by a number of psychological factors, including the aroma and taste of foods.

Blood Sampling and Analysis

Aa blood test is often prescribed by doctors to help diagnose a person's health condition. The blood sample is sent to a laboratory where technicians analyze the blood using specialized instruments and techniques. Various tests may be performed on a blood sample, including a complete blood count (CBC), which is used to detect a wide range of health disorders such as anemia, infection and leukemia, and a blood glucose test which is used to help diagnose diabetes and monitor blood glucose levels. None of the tests are conclusive in themselves but are used to help diagnose a patient's condition and determine what follow-up tests should be prescribed.

In Appendix D of his book, *The Detox Miracle Sourcebook*, Robert Morse describes how anyone can interpret the results of the blood work that a doctor has prescribed for them. It includes a description of blood types (Types A, B, AB, etc.), the meaning of red and white blood cell counts, and the limitations that the diagnostics have. It lists reference ranges for nutrients that are found in the blood. The ranges are based on analyses of blood of presumably healthy people. But the point is, it seems that the body requires nutrients to be within certain ranges for health.

According to T. Colin Campbell in his book, *Whole, Rethinking the Science of Nutrition.* the body is continually monitoring and adjusting the concentrations of nutrients in the blood to maintain the ranges it requires for health. He explains how medical and governmental understanding of nutrition is rooted in the reductionist paradigm, a way of thinking that everything can be understood through its component parts. He contends that a wholistic approach to health is what is required to understand nutrition. A wholistic approach considers how the various component parts work together, which is in line with how nature operates. Nature works in wholistic ways, with all parts working together, never with one part working on its own. This is a very important concept to understand in our journey to optimum health.

"When you're looking through a microscope, either literally or metaphorically, you can't see the big picture." - T. Colin Campbell and Howard Jacobson, *Whole, Rethinking the Science of Nutrition.*

An old saying seems to be apropos here, "You can't see the forest for the trees." We cannot see the forest when we are focusing on the trees.

Nutritionists have known for many years that the condition of the urine reveals much about the blood's condition. For example, if the urine is cloudy, the blood is likely to be cloudy too, such as when protein intake has thickened it. The pH of urine closely matches the pH of the blood, and can be used to determine the blood's pH condition. Litmus paper is a useful tool in this regard. It is another example of how we can become more our own doctor. We can test our urine's pH. Strips of litmus paper may be purchased on the Web.

If you consume alcohol at night, it is important to eat alkalizing raw plant foods before going to bed to counteract the acidic blood chemistry caused by alcoholic beverages. It will give you better, sounder sleeps.

Blood is discussed further in the chapter on "Distilled Water."

Antioxidants

Antioxidants are substances that protect the cells of the body against the effects of free radicals. Antioxidants neutralize free radicals. Antioxidants include beta-carotene, lycopene, p-coumaric acid, and vitamins A, C, and E (alpha-tocopherol), all of which are found in raw plant foods.

Free Radicals

A free radical is a molecule that with an unpaired electron. It is "free" to react "radically" with other molecules and cause cellular disruption and damage.

According to the National Cancer Institute, damage to the cells of the body caused by free radicals play an important role in the development of cancer and other serious health disorders.

Antioxidants are the body's main defenses against free radicals. They neutralize free radicals by chemically combining them with the molecules in the foods. As discussed in the chapter on "The Causes of Disease," foods that are rich in antioxidants are known to stop or reverse toxic buildup.

We should eat foods that are high in antioxidants. The foods of the raw vegan diet are rich in enzymes, nutrients and antioxidants. Whole plant foods that are particularly rich in antioxidants are listed below.

WHOLE PLANT FOODS HIGH IN ANTIOXIDANTS

Fruits – all kinds
Green leafy vegetables (Greens) -- all kinds

Vegetables – all kinds
Spices and herbs
Superfoods

It is important to eat as many antioxidant-rich foods as we can to strengthen the immune system, neutralize the poisons within the body and stop or reverse toxic buildup in the body.

Most antioxidants are destroyed by heat. While freezing seems to preserve antioxidant activity, heating adversely affects almost all antioxidants. This means, for example, that canned and jarred fruits and vegetables, which have been heat treated during refining and processing, have significantly lower levels of antioxidants than their living food counterparts. It indicates that fruits and vegetables that are fast-frozen are acceptable to eat on the raw vegan diet.

Oxidative Stress

Oxidative stress occurs when an imbalance exists between free radical activity and antioxidant activity in the body. An ordinary diet, such as the Standard American Diet, causes oxidative stress which contributes to aging and degenerative diseases. It is known that when foods contain insufficient antioxidants to counteract free radicals, the resulting imbalance can damage the DNA and the proteins and fatty tissues of the body.

Researchers have shown that mental stress creates free radicals. Radiation, environmental pollutants, such as smog, cigarette smoke, car exhaust fumes and impurities and toxins in municipal drinking water, also create free radicals.

Agricultural chemicals are known to destroy the antioxidants in crops. Therefore, it is wise to eat organic produce to maximize the antioxidants we receive from natural plant foods.

According to Dr. Michael Greger's book, How Not To Die, antioxidant supplements, such as vitamin C and beta carotene, do not work. The body needs to get its antioxidants from living plant foods.

Antioxidant Ratings

The ORAC (Oxygen Radical Absorbance Capacity) is considered a useful antioxidant rating system, although it is not the only one.

ORAC was used by the USDA until 2012, which, according to the Web, was the year USDA's Nutrient Data Laboratory (NDL) removed the ORAC Database for Selected Foods from the NDL website. It was removed due to pressure on the USDA from independent laboratories that argued that "in vitro" tests do not conclusively reflect what happens in the human body. It is uncertain whether the pressure was due to legitimate concerns or based on the biased opinion of the meat and dairy industries. However, it appears to be a somewhat specious argument since measuring the effect of antioxidants in the human body is not possible, according to papers published on the Web at the time of this writing.

Nevertheless, ORAC is still used by many nutritionists as a comparative basis for antioxidant capacity since it reflects how effectively a food or product neutralizes free radicals as measured by the degradation of a fluorescent dye. ORAC is a particularly useful measure of the antioxidant effectiveness of foods that contain complex ingredients with both slow- and fast-acting antioxidants, and also foods that have combined or synergistic effects.

ORAC ratings of various herbs and spices, taken from the Web at the time of this writing, are listed below.

SAMPLE OF ORAC ANTIOXIDANT RATINGS

Cloves, ground   314, 446

Cinnamon, ground   267, 536

Oregano, dried   200,129

Rosemary, dried   165, 280

Parsley, dried   73, 670

Many foods that are commonly eaten today, such as meat- and dairy-based foods, have, in comparison to the above values, negligible ORAC ratings, which indicates low antioxidant effectiveness. These foods include, but are not limited to, salmon with an ORAC rating of 30, eggs (20), hot dogs (300), McDonald's Crispy Chicken Sandwich (180), Little Caesar's Cheese Pizza (180), and fried chicken (50).

At the time of this writing, a complete listing of ORAC ratings of many foods is available on the following website:

https://www.cupcrfoodly.com/orac-values/

It should be noted that the ORAC rating is based on 100 grams of food. Since raw fruits and vegetables, including fresh (undried) herbs, have water content, the ORAC ratings of these foods are much lower than their dried alternatives. If this is not considered, the ORAC ratings of raw fruits and vegetables can be misleading.

When we eat living plant foods, the body is provided with all the nutrients it needs for optimum health, including Nature's own antioxidants. The body's defenses against free radicals are the greatest when we eat raw plant foods, which means the immune system is strengthened by these foods. Antioxidant supplements, such as the vitamin C and beta carotene supplements that are available today, are not good sources for the antioxidants the body needs. The raw vegan diet is the best assurance that anyone can have of getting the antioxidants needed for health.

The Food Pyramid

The United States Department of Agriculture (USDA) has issued its Food Guide Pyramid since 1992. The Guide is intended to help Americans reduce their intake of total fat and choose what and how much to eat from each of the food groups that are depicted on the pyramid. The government's involvement in the issuance of nutritional guidelines shows how far we have drifted away from the basics of proper health and nutrition.

The food pyramid is often displayed on packaged foods, such as breads. However, it is the firm conviction of many of nutritionists that the USDA Food Pyramid does not, and never has, properly reflected what is best for human health. Rather, it reflects what the food industry says is best for health.

The meat, dairy and grain businesses, which are the chief vested interests in perpetuating the Standard American Diet, have influenced federal dietary regulations for decades. It is commonly believed that these interests write the protocols of the USDA. As stated in a dietary guideline article published on the Web, "After all, what is the USDA if not the regulatory body created to ensure that the U.S. agricultural commodities (like corn, soy, and wheat) are profitable?" These interests are interested first, last and always in profits, not in human welfare.

It is well known that most of the grain produced in the world goes to feed livestock in order to supply food stores and restaurants with cold cuts and other meat products.

Most of us realize by now the power that big businesses have to make the rules. But health awareness and a knowledge of foods and nutrition give us the freedom to eat the healthier foods that are available for us to eat.

The food pyramid is not our friend. When I started searching for the answers about how foods and nutrition impact human health years ago, I was often led astray by the food pyramid because of my gullibility to accept what governmental bodies recommend should be my diet. As discussed in this book, many nutritionists, including those whose books are listed in the Bibliography, have been telling us for years that meat, dairy and grain products are harmful to human health.

The food pyramid of 1992 to 2005 (see below) shows bread, cereal, rice and pasta at the bottom, or base, of the pyramid, indicating that grain products should be the most often eaten food. However, all grains, even raw grain seeds, are starchy foods. And pasta, sweet rolls and bread are cooked foods. As discussed in this book, cooked and starchy foods are harmful to human health. For a healthy diet, the food pyramid would not have grain products as the base, nor would it include cooked foods.

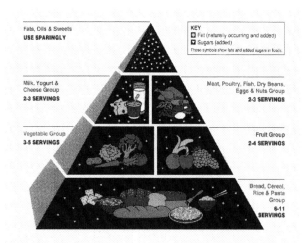

The Food Guide Pyramid from 1992 to 2005

The food pyramid of 2005 to 2011 (below), makes even less sense. It doesn't have a clearly defined base or hierarchy. It shows five food groups (grains, vegetables, fruits, milk, and meat and beans), sharing the same base. There is no one food group at the base of the pyramid. At first glance, it indicates that there is no one food group any better for health than another. It implies that you should eat a portion of each.

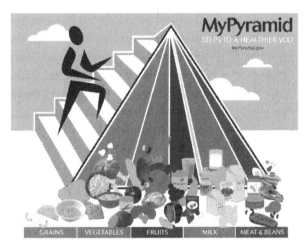

The Food Guide Pyramid from 2005 to 2011

It is not surprising that grains, milk and meat are three of the five food groups that share the base of this food pyramid. The meat, dairy and grain businesses are those with the largest vested interests in continuing the production of animal products for the Standard American Diet.

For most of us, the food pyramid of 2005 to 2011 is too confusing to be an effective dietary guideline.

The Food Pyramid has recently (2019) been superseded by MyPlate (see below), also published by the USDA. MyPlate is a depiction of a pie-shaped plate of food on a table with a drink off to one side. Five food groups, Fruits, Vegetables, Grains, Proteins and Milk, are represented.

There are no MyPlate details in the depiction to reveal what each food group consists of, but they may be accessed on the Web. For example, for Fruits, the details list as options, fresh, canned, frozen, dried, cut up or pureed. For Proteins, the details list seafood, meat, poultry and eggs, nuts, seeds and soy. The drink off to the side is milk. The dangers of eating canned food products, and most of the protein options (excepting nuts and seeds), have been discussed in this book. Also, as discussed previously, vegetables provide all the proteins needed for human health. The MyPlate design implies that we need to eat foods from all five food groups, including dairy, and in every form sold to the public.

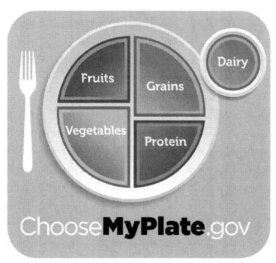

The current (2019) USDA Food Guideline

In the age of information, a food pyramid or pie plate that would really make sense would be one that would give priority to eating raw fruits and vegetables over everything else, with nuts, seeds, and water included in the design. It would not include meat- and dairy-based foods, grain products or canned foods.

However, it probably doesn't matter what the food pyramids or other depictions look like. Guidelines do not make people knowledgeable no matter how instructive they may be. Knowledge about foods and nutrition is not gained by glancing at a food pyramid or pie chart. Our current obesity epidemic, as described in the chapter on "The Causes of Disease," clearly indicates the public's failure to follow any dietary guidelines.

People make society what it is. Most people eat whatever they want as often as they want, regardless of the complications and discomforts that result. But what most people eat and how they eat does not have to be the way that we eat.

Each of us can work to produce a better society by the food choices we make every day. As mentioned previously, unless we have a knowledge of foods and nutrition, we lack the information needed on how health issues come about. Without this knowledge, we remain wholly ignorant of how to prevent diseases and other health disorders from taking root in the body, and how to cure them if they do. A knowledge of foods and nutrition enables us to make the right food choices, those that result in real health, which is health in tune with Nature.

We must learn what is best for us to eat and carefully guard our health from being destroyed by the cultural norms of the tempting world.

The Importance of Fasting

Fasting is purposely depriving the body of food, particularly food that is difficult to digest. Freshly-squeezed fruit juices may be allowed on fasts since they are easily digested in less than about 30 minutes and do not tax the enzyme reserves of the body.

For optimum health, some type of fasting, even if it is just eating less during meals, should be regularly practiced. The reason for this is that the evidence gained on fasting cures for diseases underlines the importance that foods have in causing and worsening diseased conditions. Nutritional experts believe that fasting is a significant part of any real health regimen, and many contend that optimum health cannot be achieved without it.

Fasting is drugless therapy. It can overcome practically any ailment common to humankind. The clinical evidence for this is very compelling as we shall see.

"Take food away from a sick man's stomach and you have begun, not to starve the sick man, but the disease." - George F. Pentecost.

Fasting may be new to the reader. I did not start fasting until in my later years, and only after I learned from books about how important fasting is for attaining optimum health. It may just be that the practice of fasting is, for most people, and particularly for most people in this country, an unknown quantity. How many people do you know who fast? Have you ever fasted? Have you ever skipped at least three meals in a row, and on purpose?

Many people relate fasting to a religious rite, such as Lent or Ramadan. However, fasting is one of the oldest customs of which there is any record. It has been practiced for thousands of years in many cultures as an essential part of healing whatever is wrong with the body. Fasting is referenced many times in both the Old and New Testaments of the Bible.

The purpose of fasting is to relieve the body of the great expenditure of energy that is required to digest foods. Digestion is considered by nutritionists to be the most energy-intensive process carried out in the human body. It is said that the stomach is the most over-worked organ because it never gets a break, except maybe at nights. In Western society, most of us are munching on something all of the time. Is there ever a time when your stomach is not busy digesting foods?

In the past 150 years, the scientific and clinical data obtained from fasting performed in the health clinics and sanatoriums of Europe and the US tell us what occurs in the body during a fast and how fasting enables the body to heal itself of diseases.

Dr. Ann Wigmore and others tell us that when animals get sick they instinctively abstain from all food. Can this be said about us? To a great extent, it cannot. Most people keep eating when they are sick on the mistaken belief that nourishment is needed for them to get well. Only rarely, such as in cases of acute fever, do we lose our appetite for food. Most doctors prescribe nourishment for those who are sick in hospitals, or who are otherwise under their care, and many patients force themselves to eat when the wisest thing to do would be to abstain from all food. It appears that in this context, animals are wiser than humans.

"Fasting works by self-digestion. During a fast your body intuitively will decompose and burn only the substances and tissues that are damaged, diseased or unneeded, such as abscesses, tumors, excess fat deposits, excess water and congestive wastes. Even a short fast (1 to 3 days) will accelerate elimination from your liver, kidneys, lungs, bloodstream and skin. Sometimes you will experience dramatic changes (cleansing and healing crisis) as accumulated wastes are expelled. With your first fasts you may temporarily have cleansing headaches, fatigue, body odor, breath coated tongue, mouth sores and even diarrhea as your body is cleaning house. Please be patient with your body!" - Paul C. and Patricia Bragg, *Water, The Shocking Truth That Can Save Your Life*,

Naturopathic healers and fasting professionals, including those who work in the renowned health institutes and clinics of Sweden, Germany and the US, such as the Buchinger-Wilhelmi fasting clinic in Germany, are keenly aware of how fasting can cure diseases. They witness daily the amazing results brought about by fasting cures, and consider fasting to be the most important curative measure in disease treatment.

Many health advocates and raw foodists regularly fast for days at a time, including Professor Spira (his book is listed in the Bibliography).

Clinical Evidence on Fasting Cures

A vast amount of clinical evidence has been obtained on fasting cures. It has resulted in thousands of publications attesting to the amazing power of fasting in enabling the body to heal itself of diseases and other health issues. They include case histories of "miraculous" cures, some of which are without precedent.

The results of a small sampling of the clinical evidence on fasting cures are given below. The first two are taken from Arnold Paul De Vries' book, *Therapeutic Fasting*.

1. 715 cases of disease were treated by fasting in Dr. James McEachen's sanatorium. The diseases included heart disease, cancer, high blood pressure, kidney disease, ulcers, colitis, arthritis and multiple sclerosis. Remedied or greatly improved by fasting were 29 of 33 cases of heart disease, 20 of 23 cases of ulcers, 3 of 4 cases of multiple sclerosis, 36 of 41 cases of kidney disease, 77 of 88 cases of colitis, 39 of 47 cases of arthritis and all of the cancer and high blood pressure cases.

2. 155 cases of disease, including a similar spectrum of diseases as indicated above, were treated through fasting by Dr. William L Esser. 113 cases experienced complete recovery, 31 experienced partial recovery, and the remaining 12 cases experienced no benefit. The percentage of improved or remedied cases was 92.3%.

3. Edward Hooker Dewey, M.D. in his books, *The True Science of Living* and *The No-Breakfast Plan and the Fasting Cure,* recounts how hundreds of patients, many of whom had the most distressing diseases, were completely cured of their diseases by fasting.

4. Hereward Carrington in his book, Vitality, Fasting and Nutrition, gives many testimonies of healing from people who were completely cured of their diseases, including paralysis and deafness.

5. Upton Sinclair in his book, The Fasting Cure, gives many testimonies of healing from people who were completely cured of their diseases.

6. Prostate cancer may be effectively treated by fasting as revealed in the following 2018 Web article,

https://sperlingprostatecenter.com/the-excitement-of-intermittent-fasting-and-you-thought-not-eating-was-boring/

The evidence gained from studies such as these indicates that fasting is the most effective method of remedying any disease or other ill-health condition. Can mainstream medicine make such claims? Does it have similar success rates in its attempts at curing the same diseases? Do the success rates of conventional medical doctors and hospitals even approach those that are obtained from fasting? Mainstream medical treatments, including surgery, chemotherapy and drugs, cannot match or even come close to the efficacy of fasting in curing diseases.

Those who have seen how fasting can cure diseases say:

"Fasting is the most efficient means of correcting any disease." - Dr. Adolph Mayer.

"Fasting is like surgery without a lancet. It cuts away the superfluous and spares what is healthy." - Erwin Hof.

"Arthritis and related diseases are usually speedily remedied by fasting, with gradual disappearance of the severe pains and swelling and the complete or partial absorption of the deformity by autolysis, providing complete ossification of the joint is not present. Fasts of one to four weeks usually alleviate arthritis, with longer fasts being employed if deformities are present." - Arnold Paul De Vries, *Therapeutic Fasting*.

"The fast is to me the key to eternal youth, the secret of perfect and permanent health. I would not take anything in all the world for my knowledge of it. It is Nature's safety valve, an automatic protection system against disease." - Upton Sinclair, *The Fasting Cure*.

For more details, the reader is referred to the books in the Bibliography by Arnold Ehret, Paavo O. Airola, Herbert M. Shelton, Arnold Paul De Vries, Edward Hooker Dewey, Upton Sinclair, Paul C. and Patricia Bragg, and Kristine Nolfi.

Unlike conventional medical methods of disease treatment that suppress one symptom only to create others, fasting helps all the organs and tissues of the body equally, with no part being helped more than another, and no part being helped at the expense of another. Fasting works on the entire body.

Whenever a cure for a disease is effected and the hand of the destroyer is stayed, it should be headline news in the media and big news in the medical profession, even if it is accomplished outside the accepted norms and teachings of conventional medicine. But how are fasting cures treated by the media or looked upon by mainstream medicine? With disdain and nonacceptance. Why? Because fasting cures do not conform to the modus operandi of the mainstream medical profession.

If mainstream medicine, in its efforts to cure diseases, could even come close to the success rates of fasting cures, it would be such a boon to civilization that it would likely eclipse all of the technological breakthroughs that have occurred in the last 120 years.

T. Colin Campbell and Howard Jacobson, in their book *Whole: Rethinking the Science of Nutrition,* describe in detail the numerous ways in which the medical industry has sacrificed health and the curing of disease for ever-increasing profits.

"Health information is controlled, and has been for a long time, by interests that are not in alignment with the common good – industries that care much more about their profit than our health.

And those industries feel deeply threatened by the possibility of mass adoption of a plant-based diet." - T. Colin Campbell and Howard Jacobson, *Whole: Rethinking the Science of Nutrition.*

Imagine, if you will, that the next time you visited a doctor, he or she advised you not to take standard medical treatments, such as medication, for your ailment, but to perform a fast. Imagine what a shock that would be to your sensibilities. But don't worry, based on the past two hundred years of standard medical practice, it is not likely to happen in our lifetime.

Despite the prejudice that mainstream medicine seems to have against fasting cures in preference to their own methods of disease treatment, the facts continue to speak for themselves. Fasting allows the body to remove the causes of an ill-health condition rather than mask its symptoms. Healing occurs naturally when the internal energy required for digestion is turned off and is made available for bodily healing and regeneration, and when, as a result of these things, it sufficiently purges itself of toxic wastes.

The body is the greatest healing machine ever. It only requires the right conditions to accomplish what it alone knows how to do. When a person fasts, food intake is stopped and the entire digestive system, including all the major organs of the body, takes a very needed physiological rest. It is this rest that allows the body to focus more on self-cleansing and on whatever needs to be healed.

During a fast, the body is amply supplied with food from within, from its stored food reserves. The food reserves of the body are so vast that death by starvation does not occur in a matter of days, but months, which is typically much longer than the average time required for healing and recovery from a fasting cure.

A Christian Diet

Francoise Wilhelmi de Toledo, in her book, *Therapeutic Fasting: The Buchinger Amplius Method*, states that a person can live on body fat for up to 40 days without suffering any harm.

There are numerous references to fasting in the Bible. Two of the most memorable fasts are those of Moses and Jesus. Both fasts were for 40 days and 40 nights (i.e., 40 complete days). Moses's fast was before he received the Ten Commandments. Jesus' fast was before He began His ministry. Many people look on these fasts as curiosities rather than facts. Some attribute them to the divine power that both Moses and Jesus had, which, of course, is the same as saying that their fasts were miracles which would not be possible for normal people under normal circumstances.

But saying that long duration fasts were, or are, miracles is refuted by the clinical evidence we have of people fasting for very long periods of time. Arnold Ehret, for example, fasted for 49 days, which was the world's record at the time. Dr. Kristine Nolfi and Dr. Wilhelmi de Toledo in their books tell us that fasts of more than 60 days have been performed in their clinics to cure diseases.

In Jesus's day, the Pharisees fasted twice a week so that others could see them in want and realize from their outward signs how religious they were. Their purpose in fasting was to gain honor from men, and Jesus condemned them for it.

Jesus must have been a thin man. No one can perform even a relatively short fast without losing a lot of body fat, as my own experiences with fasting have proven. He may have been husky as a carpenter prior to His ministry, but, in my opinion, He was a thin man later on

To many of the saints of old, fasting was a way of life, something they believed was necessary for proper living, purification and acceptance before God. They believed that it made the soul clear and light for the reception of divine truth. For example, in New Testament times, fasting was thought to be necessary for purifying the body (the temple of the Holy Spirit), and for earnest prayer.

Is there any truth in these things from what we know about the effects of fasting on spirituality? Yes! We know that fasting cleanses and purifies the body, freeing it of its burden of toxic wastes and digestion, and that this enhances one's spirituality.

The book, *The Essene Gospel of Peace, Book One*, which is described in a separate chapter of this book, and from which I have included a number of quotations for this book, provides many insights on fasting. I highly recommend it to anyone who is interested in seriously curing a health disorder or disease.

The Reluctance to Fast

In my opinion, although I hope I am wrong, fasting will never be a popular cure for disease or any other health disorder because it involves too much self-denial. In addition, a knowledge of fasting is required to go forward with the practice.

Many people today do not want to go without food for any length of time, much less for the time it takes to do a legitimate fast. I believe it has much to do with our eating habits. But there's also the hubris connected with eating in this country, the pride of having a surfeit of food. We have more food than our population needs, or can use, and in such variety and availability that it is the envy of the world. So, why pass up the opportunity to indulge while you can? It speaks of the "eat, drink and be merry, for tomorrow we die" attitude exposed in the Bible. It speaks of the dog-eat-dog, haves-and-haves-not world in which we live. It also suggests many of the attitudes that were prevalent in the ancient Roman Empire before its decline and fall.

Another reason that people do not want to fast is because they do not want to miss out on the pleasures of eating, and, in particular, eating foods that stimulate the pleasure centers of the brain, such as sugary foods, meat and dairy foods, and salty, oily and/or greasy foods.

But regardless of how much we may like to eat, the fact remains that eating is one of the major causes of pain and suffering in the world. By consuming foods that are bad for us, and maintaining improper eating habits, we reap the consequences of ill-health and disease. However, if we give up harmful pacifiers for the brain and palate, and focus on foods that truly nourish us, foods that are needed by the body for cellular reconstruction and health, and do not contain toxins that end up being stored in the body's tissues and joints, then these harmful consequences can be avoided. Not only that, but a daily diet of raw fruits and vegetables sharpens the taste buds so flavors we never knew existed before can be enjoyed.

Fasting should be more acceptable and easier for those who are already accustomed to self-denial, repentance and humility.

Other Considerations

Wallace D. Wattles in his book, *Health Through New Thought and Fasting*, states that all overeating comes from the false belief that strength is gained by eating food. The chapter on "Vitality" explains this in more detail.

Conventional wisdom and the claims of the food industry insist that we need high protein food to be strong and heathy. But this appears to be very misleading and wrong. As explained elsewhere in this book, raw plant foods, which are not high protein foods, provide all the protein needed for a healthy, active life. Also, the protein in plant foods is not the hard to digest protein of meat and dairy products. As discussed previously in the chapter on "The Causes of Disease," animal protein is complex protein that must be broken down before it can be assimilated by the body. The breaking down process results in the generation of an excessive amount of uric acid, which is known to cause uric acid crystals to form in the body that cause kidney stones and gout.

Wattles challenges us to prove conventional wisdom wrong by eating natural plant foods exclusively, cutting out one meal a day, and taking 24-36-hour fasts once a week for 4-5 months. This will be further explored in the chapter on "Vitality."

I followed Mr. Wattles' advice and can testify that it makes a big difference in the energy levels and feelings of well-being that I have. I skip breakfasts entirely, never eating anything until later in the mornings.

Clinical studies on fasting prove that a person does not become weaker by fasting, but that the strength of the body increases without foods, especially high protein foods. This is the opposite of what we have been led to expect, but it is true.

"Contrary to popular belief, you don't get weakened or depleted by fasting. On the contrary, fasting will strengthen the body in many ways. The stomach and digestive tract will receive a rest and will be strengthened by fasting." - Paavo O. Airola, N.D., *There is a Cure for Arthritis.*

Fasts longer than a week are typically recommended to allow the body to cure diseases. In general, the worse the disease or health condition, the longer the fast should be to correct the situation.

Note: For fasts over a week long, it is recommended that the aspirant seek the supervision of a physician or fasting professional.

How to Fast

Short-term fasts, typically of no more than 4 days' duration, may be done at home without the supervision or expense of a fasting professional. You can learn about them by reading books on fasting, such as the books on fasting that are listed in the Bibliography, including Paul C. and Patricia Bragg's book, *The Miracle of Fasting*.

It is commonly observed by those who fast regularly that after about the third day there is no longer a feeling of hunger.

Fasting is not that difficult. You get used to it very soon. It does wonders not only for the body but also for the soul. When I fast, I like to read about fasting and think about how much energy is being conserved from the high-energy demands of digestion and is being used for deep bodily cleansing and healing. Drinking pure distilled water, with or without herbal teas (such as chamomile and lavender), fills the stomach and quells hunger. I typically fast every morning, and more often when I sense the need for it. It is a wonderful learning and growing experience.

You should fast when you can detect your body's signals to fast. It is then that you should fast. However, if you have a serious health condition, then you should jump into fasting right away.

The first fast is a real learning experience, and there will be hunger pangs because of eating habits. But Nature knows best. Fight the 4-6 meals a day habit and try fasting whenever you are ready for it. You won't die, and it will be a new experience for you, a richly rewarding experience that only you will know about.

"It is requisite that men should live up to the simplicity of nature, which teaches us to be content with little, and accustom ourselves to eat no more than is absolutely necessary to support life, remembering that all excess causes disease and leads to death." - Luigi Cornaro, *How to Live 100 Years, or Discourses on the Sober Life*.

You should have a goal or objective for the fast, such as to remedy a health issue or fight a disease. If you think about the goal when fasting, it will help you to complete the fast.

I try to fast often to give my digestive organs a break. The longest duration fast for me was 5 days, during which time I ingested only distilled water or herbal teas in distilled water. I broke the fast because I didn't see any need for prolonging it since I had already been on the raw vegan diet for some time and enjoyed good health by the continued self-cleansing that an exclusive diet of raw plant foods provides. However, whenever my body tells me to abstain from foods, I will fast.

I recommend that fasting be practiced regularly like all other aspects of the raw vegan diet. In my opinion, all raw vegans should perform at least a 2-day fast periodically, drinking only distilled water or herbal teas in distilled water during those two days. When the time is right, which is typically when the body has been on the self-cleansing diet for a year or more, we should learn how to fast.

A type of fasting that may be practiced at every meal is eating less during meals, such as ending meals when we are two-thirds full. It's a skill that you can learn which promotes genuine health. Fasting produces a profound and beneficial effect on the nerves as well as the psyche and health of the individual.

"Your fasting is always pleasing in the eyes of the angels of God. So give heed to how much you have eaten when your body is sated, and always eat less by a third." - Attributed to Jesus, *The Essene Gospel of Peace, Book One.*

One of the things fasting does is make us more cognizant of what we are putting into the body. It makes us more aware of the quality and quantity of the foods we eat. It also makes us more aware of what food combinations are doing us harm.

I recommend the books on fasting by Herbert M. Shelton, Paul C. and Patricia Bragg, Arnold Ehret, Paavo Airola and Professor Spira (see Bibliography). They cover most aspects of fasting and describe everything one needs to know about how best to perform fasts, especially the first fast. These books clearly reveal that fasting should be a way of life in order to escape the many of the ways of death.

The big myth is that we have to eat a lot to be healthy.

Each of the above-recommended books on fasting has recommendations on how long one should fast. Take Paul C. Bragg's book for example. He recommends progressing as follows (my remarks are added):

1. At first, do a weekly fast of 24-36 hours. You learn a great deal on the very first fast. Fasting gets easier as you continue.

2. After maintaining the weekly fast, do a 3-4 day fast in addition to the weekly fast. These fasts are very effective in dissolving deep-rooted, accumulated toxins.

3. After fasting as recommended above for about 6 months, add in a 7 day fast.

4. After about a year of continuing the above fasting program, do a 10 day fast.

Arnold Ehret in his book, *The Mucusless Diet Healing System*, states that the most exact and unerring diagnosis of a person's overall health condition is how they respond to a short fast. The more quickly a person feels worse during a short fast, the greater are his encumbrances and the worse is his overall health condition.

Ehret recommends starting at first with the no-breakfast plan, then following up with a 24-hour fast, learning as you go. Then gradually increase up to 3, 4 or 5-day fasts, while between fasting providing and rebuilding the body with the best raw materials, such as found in mucusless foods (raw fresh fruit, leafy greens and non-starchy vegetables). Such an intermittent fasting program will gradually improve and regenerate the blood and dissolve and eliminate deposited wastes from the deepest tissues of the body.

"All the vitality and all the energy I have comes to me because my body is purified by fasting." - Mahatma Gandhi.

Fasting assists the body's self-cleansing process which helps us attain optimum health. When the body is sufficiently cleansed of the poisonous waste materials that have accumulated in it from years of wrong eating, then comes true health, health as you may have never experienced it before. We need to use fasting, as well as colonics and enemas, to purify our bodies of the filth that has accumulated in them from years of wrong eating.

"Renew yourselves and fast. For I tell you truly, that Satan and his plagues may only be cast out by fasting and prayer. Go by yourself and fast alone, and show your fasting to no man. The living God shall see it and great shall be your reward. For I tell you truly, except you fast, you shall never be freed from the power of Satan and from all diseases that come from Satan." - Attributed to Jesus, *The Essene Gospel of Peace, Book One.*

Each fast is a new adventure, a break from the almost constant digestion that occurs in the body, a time when all the organs of the body take a very needed break, and, just as importantly, a break from the daily routines and behavior patterns we all strive to maintain.

Before your first fast, I recommend changing your diet to the living plant food raw vegan diet. You can jump into the diet directly, or transition to it from whatever diet you may be on, as discussed in the chapter on "Transitioning to the God-given Diet."

Fasting causes a marked improvement in an ill-health condition. But the efficacy of fasting in curing ailments depends on the individual's eating habits and how long they have been practiced. It also depends on the duration of the fast. According to fasting care professionals, relief from excruciating pain, such as from rheumatoid arthritis, can be had within only a few days of beginning a fast, but longer fasts are often required to completely eradicate the disease.

"However, this kind does not go out except by prayer and fasting." - Jesus in the Bible, Matt. 17:21.

Persistence, willpower and patience are often required for natural cures to be effective. Fasting is one of the ways they can be learned.

If anyone could reap the benefits of fasting without going out of their way and exerting effort, then everyone would be routinely fasting for their health. But all things are given to us at the price of labor.

Learn about fasting and you will reap its benefits. Do nothing and you will reap the consequences of inaction when action may be just what is needed in your life.

Proper Eating Habits

"We are not what we eat but what we assimilate" - Paavo O. Airola.

Those who wolf, gulp or bolt down their foods are prone to digestive discomforts and disorders, including heartburn and stomachache to mention only two. Many regularly resort to quick remedies, such as antacids, aspirin and similar drugs. According to the Web, at least $2 billion are spent yearly in the US alone on antacids, and $10 billion worldwide. That's a lot of indigestion!

In addition, many people eat compulsively, often consuming food throughout the day whenever they feel like it, whether they're hungry or not. Compulsive eating can be out of habit or because of job-prescribed or tradition-prescribed meal times. If we eat food when we are not hungry, the body is not ready for the food.

These habits are damaging to the human system, and the damage gets worse the more they are practiced. They cannot produce vibrant health because the foods cannot be properly digested and assimilated by the body. Not only do they cause digestive difficulties, but they cause sluggishness and grogginess, general fatigue and various illnesses. An old saying is:

One quarter of what you eat keeps you alive. The other quarter keeps your doctor alive.

Proper eating habits are prescribed by Nature. Food must be eaten in such a way that the full powers of the digestive system are employed. In addition, every ounce of food that passes through the body that is not actually needed by the body is a tax on the body's vital powers, a waste of vital energy.

To avoid these complications and more, most of us need to modify our eating habits.

Digestion occurs primarily in two ways, mechanical digestion and chemical digestion.

Mechanical digestion occurs as the teeth grind and masticate foods. Chewing breaks down food into smaller particles which allows them to be better digested. An old saying is: "Chew your food, your stomach has no teeth."

Chemical digestion begins in the mouth through saliva. The process of chewing activates the flow of saliva. If the mouth does not water during a meal then the body is not ready for the food, and digestion of that food will be hindered. Some nutritionists claim that food well-salivated is practically half-digested before it gets to the stomach. Many raw foodists recommend chewing food until it is liquified in the mouth. In addition, when whole plant foods are eaten, the enzymes in these foods assist in the chemical digestive process.

Two thousand years ago, Asclepiades of Greece understood that particles of food are a main cause of indigestion. If the particles were small, digestion would follow its normal course, but if the particles were too big, indigestion would occur.

"The chief function of today's cook is to prepare soft pap for the adult, so that little or no chewing is required. Meats are pounded or ground and vegetables cooked to make them easy to swallow with a minimum of chewing; breads are made to be swallowed with very little preliminary mastication; potatoes are mashed, cereals soaked and fruits stewed, so that the muscles of the jaw get very little exercise and the food gets very little saliva. There is no real pleasure in such eating." - Dr. Herbert M. Shelton, *Health for the Millions*.

To get the most of foods, and produce the kind of health we all want and need, the following eating habits should be practiced at every meal.

1. All foods should be eaten slowly, and chewed thoroughly. If you are very hungry before eating, you should still slow down on the eating or the foods will be wolfed or bolted down with little chewing taking place.

2. Do not overeat. This is the cardinal rule to master if you want to obtain optimum health. As discussed in the chapter on "The God-given Diet," it may be best for us to eat no more than 2 quarts of food per day. The best advice I can offer is the same as that of many others, which is to leave the table when you are 2/3 full. This has often been difficult for me to learn, but I found that when I practiced it everything changed for the better on my journey to optimum health. What it amounts to is eating only as much as your system actually needs. Only you can determine that. It may take a while to learn, but it is all part of the journey.

"Every individual should, as a general rule, restrain himself to the smallest quantity which he finds from careful investigation, enlightened experience and observation will fully meet the alimentary wants of his system, knowing that whatsoever is more than this is evil." - Dr. Sylvester Graham.

3. Adhere to the proper food combination laws (see the chapter on "Proper Food Combinations.")

4. Make sure fruits are ripe before eating them. How to tell when fruits are ready to be eaten was discussed previously.

5. Enjoy your food! If food is not enjoyed it cannot be efficiently digested. It is why I recommend using a raw vegan dipping sauce for raw vegetables, at least until the food can be enjoyed au naturel, without sauce.

6. If emotionally strung out or upset about something before eating, then skip the meal. Studies have shown that fear, anxiety, tension and anger constrict the entire digestive system and dry up the digestive juices.

7. Limit water or other fluid intake during a meal. It only dilutes the digestive juices that are needed for proper digestion. Drink any liquids at least 1/2 hour before, and typically no sooner than 1 hour after a meal. Protein and fat meals require the longest times to pass through the stomach (up to 4 hours), so adjust the consumption of liquids after the meal accordingly.

8. Eat to live, instead of live to eat. This was the dictum of Socrates, the most exemplary of the Greek philosophers. It represents the tried and tested way of health attained by the Greeks during the Golden Age of Athens.

"The rest of the world lives to eat, but I eat to live." - Socrates (470-399 B.C.).

Doing these things, or even only five of them, greatly assists in obtaining the health and vigor we are all seeking.

The Good and Bad About Salt

Salt (sodium chloride) is essential to life. The Romans paid their troops in salt, hence the word "salary." Our bodies need salt, but there are different kinds of salt and some have proven to be harmful to the body.

Robert O. Young and Shelley R. Young, in their book, *The pH Miracle*, describe the differences between what they consider to be "bad salt" and "good salt." "Bad salt" is common table salt, the salt that is widely used in homes and restaurants in America and throughout the world, and is the salt commonly added to refined and processed foods. Let's talk about table salt before discussing the "good salt."

Nutritional experts and even members of the medical profession have implicated table salt with the high incidence of high blood pressure and kidney problems in the Western world. Table salt is unnatural, highly-refined salt that has been heat treated to very high temperatures which alters the chemical structure of the salt. The salt is then bleached white and combined with anti-caking agents, fluoride, dextrose, aluminum hydroxide (to improve its pour-ability) and preservatives. Aluminum is widely recognized as a neurotoxin and a potential cause of Alzheimer's disease. An easy way to recognize refined salt is its bleached white color.

As explained in *The pH Miracle*, many of the additives in table salt, such as those listed above, are not required to be listed on food labels, including the food labels on canned, bottled and jarred (refined and processed) foods and the food labels on packages of salt. These labels typically just list "salt" as an ingredient.

The Web has some good articles about the health hazards of table salt. For example, search on "common table salt health" or "table salt poison."

F. Batmanghelidj, M.D, in his book, *Your Body's Many Cries for Salt*, states that the salt we use should be unrefined sea salt.

Jacques de Langre in his book, *Sea Salt's Hidden Powers*, states that refined and processed salt has an altered chemical structure and lacks the electrolytic positive and negative charge properties that natural sea salt possesses.

Many products with "sea salt" as an ingredient actually contain refined sea salt, not unrefined, natural sea salt. I wish I had known that years ago when I used "iodized sea salt" on my foods. *The pH Miracle* states that 89% of all sea salt commercially sold has been refined and processed, that is, its chemical structure has been altered by extreme heat and chemicals have been added. Like table salt, refined sea salt is always bleached white in color. The sea salt I was using for years was bright white in color.

Natural sea salt, the kind that comes from evaporating sea water by the heat of the sun, is not refined, meaning that it has not been heat treated by modern refining techniques, and it does not contain man-made additives. It is not blanched white like refined salts, but has a natural grayish or pinkish cast to it.

There are several commercially available natural sea salts to choose from. An example is Celtic Sea Salt, which is a North Atlantic Ocean sun-evaporated salt. It contains over 80 minerals and is considered a full-spectrum natural sea salt. Other brands include Pink Himalayan Sea Salt and Real Salt, both of which are mined from salt deposits in the earth that apparently were formed by the Biblical Flood. Pink Himalayan sea salt comes from

Pakistan. and Real Salt comes from Utah. You can learn more about these salts on the Web.

F. Batmanghelidj in his book referenced above states that there are hidden "miracles" in unrefined sea salt. These include:

• Extracting excess acidity from the cells of the body, particularly the brain cells.

• Preserving the serotonin and melatonin levels in the brain.

• It is vital for the communication and information processing of nerve cells.

• Salt and water perform natural antioxidant duties and clear toxic waste from the body.

• Maintaining muscle tone and strength, reduces stress and emotional disorders and assists sleep.

"A salt-free diet is utterly stupid." - F. Batmanghelidj, *Your Body's Many Cries for Salt.*

One of the leading experts on foods and nutrition in the world today is undoubtedly David Wolfe. Some of his books are listed in the Bibliography. There is probably no one who has eaten as many different kinds of raw plant foods, or has used as many different kinds of natural sea salt, as he. For additional information about sea salt, see David Wolfe's You Tube videos on salt.

Arnold Ehret, in his book, *The Mucusless Diet Healing System*, states that salt is a very good mucus dissolver.

Despite all the good that is reported about using natural sea salt, the fact remains that sea salt is an inorganic salt. Most nutritionists assert that the body cannot effectively utilize inorganic minerals of any kind, such as inorganic iodine, sodium, calcium, iron, phosphorus, magnesium, etc. They also assert that inorganic minerals not eliminated by normal bodily processes get stored in the body's tissues and joints. Nutritionists, including those referenced in this book, firmly believe that we should get all our minerals from plants.

"Inorganic minerals are not completely purged from the body by the kidneys and other body organs -- only a portion of them are. The rest accumulate in the body tissues and joints. Over time, this accumulation of inorganic minerals results in various degenerative diseases, including arthritis. This accumulation is also said to be the cause of a general enfeebled rigidity called "old age." - N. W. Walker, *Water Can Undermine Your Health*.

As discussed previously, plants transform inorganic minerals from the soil and also the ocean into organic form that is easily assimilated by the body. Organic salt is contained in vegetables, including sea vegetables, and is what the body needs for health.

"The bottom line is this – no matter where or how on earth it comes from, if salt is not first transformed by plants from inorganic sodium into organic sodium, it can't be properly absorbed by the body!" - Paul C. Bragg, *Water, The Shocking Truth That Can Save Your Life*.

On a whole plant food diet. there is no lack of mineral salts for electrolyte health. If additional salt is desired because of worries about not getting enough salt, then you should use natural, unrefined sea salt.

Dr. Ann Wigmore in her book, *Be Your Own Doctor*, states that inorganic salts can get deposited in the joints of the body and cause arthritis. She healed herself of arthritis by eliminating table salt from her diet and going on a whole plant food diet.

As explained in N.W. Walker's book, *The Natural Way to Vibrant Health,* sea water has all the mineral elements in colloidal (liquid) form. He tells us how he used sea water on his foods with no adverse reactions. It appears that if water is added to natural sea salt and the salt is allowed to dissolve, it would return its minerals to colloidal form as they exist in sea water.

The body needs electrolytes for health. I have been using natural sea salt, such as Celtic Sea Salt and Real Salt, on my vegetables for years without seeing any ill effects. I believe that it is due to it being readily assimilated by the body.

The National Academy of Medicine (NAM) recommends limiting salt intake to 1500 mg per day, or about half a teaspoon per day.

I hope that this chapter has provided useful information regarding this important and controversial topic. If you decide to use salt, you should use natural, unrefined sea salt, and use it sparingly.

Distilled Water

"Pure distilled water is truly God's greatest gift to us, a source of life and health." - Paul C. Bragg.

Drinking distilled water has received a bad rap over the years. This chapter explains why distilled water is, in fact, beneficial to human health and should be the water of choice for all who strive for optimum health.

Contrary to popular belief/misconception, our blood is not comprised of regular water. Human blood is comprised of about 78% fluid, and 90% of it is distilled water. According to nutritional experts, including Dr. N. W. Walker, Paul C. Bragg, and Dr. Allen E. Banik (who spent most of his life researching the effects of water on the human body), we do not need regular water to sustain health, and, more significantly, regular water is harmful to human health. This startling contention is explored in this chapter.

As we progress in our understanding of foods and nutrition, many of the things that humankind has taken for granted throughout the centuries may be exposed as untruths or falsehoods.

Regular water, which includes tap or faucet water, drinking-fountain water, spring, well, river and lake water, is water that has been in contact with the rocks and soil. It also includes filtered water since minerals in regular water are in solution[10] and do not get filtered out. What we normally refer to as "water" includes all of the aforementioned types. They contain inorganic minerals, such as lime (calcium), sodium, iron, phosphorus, magnesium,

---

[10] The most commonly dissolved minerals are sodium, calcium, magnesium, potassium, chloride, bicarbonate and sulfate.

etc., that have been collected from the rocks or soil that the water has been in contact with.

Distilled water has no inorganic minerals and is devoid of chlorination and fluoridation, heavy metals and pesticides. It is the type of water most compatible with the human body's cells. It is entirely safe for human consumption, and ideally meets the needs of the body.

Also, contrary to popular belief/misconception, distilled water does not leach out minerals that have become part of the body's cells. This in confirmed in Robert Morse's book, *The Detox Miracle Sourcebook,* which states that distilled water dissolves inorganic minerals that are lodged in the tissues and joints of the body, and greatly assists in removing them from the body, but it does not cause minerals that are part of the body's cells to be leached out. Dr. N. W. Walker in his book, *Water Can Undermine Your Health*, states the following:

"It is virtually impossible for distilled water to separate minerals which have become an integral part of the cells and tissues of the body. Distilled water collects only the minerals which remain in the body, minerals discarded from natural water and from the cells, the minerals which the natural water originally collected from its contact with the earth and the rocks. Such minerals, having been rejected by the cells of the body are of no constructive value. On the contrary, they are debris which distilled water is capable of picking up and eliminating from the system." - Dr. N. W. Walker, *Water Can Undermine Your Health*.

Again, distilled water cannot leach out minerals that have become part of the body's cells. What it can do is leach out excess minerals that are deposited in the joints and tissues of the body, minerals that the body could not properly utilize.

"Distilled water acts as a solvent in the body. It dissolves food substances so they can be assimilated and taken into every cell. It dissolves inorganic mineral substances lodged in tissues of the body so that such substances can be eliminated in the process of purifying the body. Distilled water is the greatest solvent on earth, the only one that can be taken into the body without damage to the tissues. By its continued use, it is possible to dissolve inorganic minerals, acid crystals, and all the other waste products of the body without injuring tissues." - Dr. Allen E. Banik, *The Choice is Clear.*

Organic minerals are the minerals we get from eating plants. Plants convert the inorganic minerals found in the water that they take up from the soil into a readily usable-by-the-body organic form. Organic minerals are not deposited in the tissues and joints of the body but are utilized by the cells of the body for their regeneration.

Distilled water is regular, hard water that has been condensed after the water is boiled. Distillation is the most effective method of purifying water. The minerals stay behind because they are not volatile, and the condensed steam is pure of minerals, bacteria, viruses and physical impurities. Even rain water is not as pure as distilled water since it contains impurities picked up by the rain from the air.

Since the time that municipal water was first chlorinated, it has been maintained by many that drinking regular water, the water that originates from streams and lakes, which includes municipal recycled water, mineral waters and bottled waters, is good for health because it has minerals the body needs. However, according to many nutritionists, inorganic minerals that are contained in regular water should not be put into the human body.

"There is only one way you can purify your body and help to eliminate your chronic aging diseases and that is through the miracle of distilled water." - Dr. Allen E. Banik, *The Choice is Clear*.

In addition to lacking inorganic minerals, distilled water is totally lacking in dangerous metals and chemicals that are found in today's drinking and bottled waters.

Paul and Patricia Bragg, in their book *Water, The Shocking Truth That Can Change Your Life,* state that the tap water we use for cooking, bathing and drinking can be responsible for many ailments because of the addition of harmful chemicals such as sodium fluoride and chlorine. The book explains the dangers of these chemicals. The authors further state that distilled water is the only water we should drink, not only because it removes inorganic mineral deposits and toxins from the joints of the body, but because it helps remove cholesterol and fat.

"Inorganic minerals, toxic chemicals, fluoride and contaminants can pollute, clog up and even turn tissues to stone throughout your body, causing pain, illness and even premature death!" - Paul C. Bragg, *Water, The Shocking Truth That Can Save Your Life*.

For similar reasons, Dr. N. W. Walker, in his many books, states that distilled water should be used for cooking and drinking.

"Distilled water is always the safest to drink. As regular water may leave deposits of calcium and other unwanted minerals in the blood circulation, these may find their way into the endocrine gland system with disastrous results which might never be attributed to these unusable minerals as the cause." - Norman W. Walker, *Water Can Undermine Your Health*.

Some people have purchased reverse osmosis water filtration units for under-the-sink home use to purify their faucet water for drinking or cooking purposes. In the reverse osmosis process, water is purified by forcing a portion of the faucet water through a semi-permeable membrane. The process removes a high percentage of the dissolved solids as well as other contaminants from the water. However, Dr. Allen E. Banik, in his book, *The Choice is Clear*, explains why reverse osmosis water is not preferable to distilled water, in the following excerpt:

"While the result [of reverse osmosis] often approaches the purity of distilled water. the degree of purity in any case varies widely, depending on the types and conditions of the equipment used, much as with filter equipment, and the effectiveness lessens with use, sometimes drastically!" - Dr. Allen E. Banik, *The Choice is Clear*.

The advantages of drinking distilled water are many as described above. From my researching, I did not find any disadvantages except for what appears on websites. For the websites that were polled for this information, I did not find any that supported the claims of the nutritionists that have been cited in this chapter. Once again, this exemplifies the disconnect that exists between the truths about foods and nutrition versus the claims on popular media.

I have been drinking distilled water for years with absolutely no ill effects. I switched from hard, faucet and bottle waters to distilled water when I read the books that describe the health benefits of drinking distilled water. I find its taste to be much better than faucet water or bottled waters, and I can testify to the positive difference it makes in my health.

My recommendation is that everyone on the raw vegan diet switch to drinking distilled water for their health. The next time you are shopping for bottled water, pick up a gallon of distilled water instead. At the time of this writing, distilled water was selling for about eighty cents per gallon at retail stores like Wal-Mart.

Within the first month of drinking distilled water, I noticed a marked increase in my thirst for the water. Previously, it seemed that I never drank very much water and I never liked the taste of it when I drank it. But now, I love the taste of water in its purist form, with its thirst-quenching ability as a bonus. Distilled water is, for me, a truly rewarding experience. There is something about distilled water and the actions it performs on the body that are very remarkable. Distilled water is what I believe the body craves.

It is said that the older we get the more we lose our ability to sense thirst. As a result, our bodies become more and more dehydrated as we continue to age, without us being able to recognize it. This chronic dehydration can cause serious health problems.

"Chronic and persistently increasing dehydration is the root cause of almost all currently encountered diseases of the human body." - F. Batmanghelidj, M.D, *Your Body's Many Cries for Water.*

What has changed my life more than anything else in recent years has been switching to the raw vegan diet and drinking distilled water.

Longevity

Alchemists, scientists and laymen throughout history have tried to discover the secrets of longevity, or a long life. It was once believed that all one had to do was to find the "Elixir of Life," which was thought to be a certain food or mixture of foods that would bestow eternal youth on its possessor.

The Holy Scriptures appear to be the origin of the belief that there once was an Elixir of Life. In Genesis 1:29, God gave to mankind a diet consisting of whole plant foods, which is best described as the raw vegan diet. But there were two trees in the Garden of Eden that had special fruit; one was the tree of good and evil, and the other was the tree of life, a tree that would make man live forever.

Genesis 2:9:
"And out of the ground the Lord God made every tree grow that is pleasant to the sight and good for food. The tree of life was also in the midst of the garden, and the tree of the knowledge of good and evil."

Genesis 3:22:
"Then the Lord God said, "Behold, the man has become like one of Us, to know good and evil. And now, lest he put out his hand and take also of the tree of life, and eat, and live forever --.""

Genesis 3:24:
"So He drove out the man; and He placed cherubim at the east of the garden of Eden, and a flaming sword which turned every way, to guard the way to the tree of life."

Many seekers of long life have wondered what kind of food grew on the Tree of Life. As far as we know, no one has succeeded in identifying it or what is probably the same thing, the Elixir of Life. But sometimes beliefs are hard to dispel, especially when they are based on truth.

Everyone wants to live longer, whether for putting things to right or for enjoyment. However, not everyone knows how to go about ensuring their longevity.

One of the great contributors to our understanding of how to live a long life was Luigi Cornaro, a nobleman who lived in Italy during the fifteenth and sixteenth centuries. His remarkable books include *Sure Methods of Attaining a long and Healthful Life, The Surest Method of Correcting an Infirm Constitution*, and *How to Live 100 Years, or Discourses on the Sober Life*. The books are listed in the Bibliography.

The term that Cornaro used in his books to describe how to attain long life through optimum health was "sobriety." By sobriety he meant the following:

"Sobriety is reduced to two things, quality and quantity. The first consists in avoiding food or drinks which are found to disagree with the stomach. The second, to avoid taking more than the stomach can easily digest." - Luigi Cornaro, *How to Live 100 Years, or Discourses on the Sober Life*.

According to his books, Cornaro ate very sparingly each and every day of his life, after curing himself in his 40s of maladies that his doctors said would soon cause his death. In his later years he never overate but always under-ate.

A Christian Diet

As discussed in the chapter on "The Foods We Should Eat and Why," immediately after the Flood, when animal food was permitted to be eaten, the average human lifespan fell from about 900 years to about 400 years. Today, according to the latest worldwide statistics, the average human lifespan is 72 years. What does this indicate? It indicates a slow decline in human longevity based on a departure from the God-given diet.

Luigi Cornaro lived to 102. What does it tell us about the importance of reducing the quantity of food that we eat, as well as fasting between meals which he obviously did by eating so sparingly? According to his books, Cornaro never needed spectacles (glasses), his hearing remained unimpaired, and he could climb hills effortlessly until he died. And he kept his mind sharp by learning new things.

In the last two hundred years, many investigators have studied extended human lifespans by visiting various cultures of the world. They have tried to ascertain why certain peoples lived longer than others. They have performed clinical studies and determined that the centenarians (those who were at least 100 years old) had the following things in common.

- They were moderate or light eaters
- They ate very little butter or salt
- They ate little, if any, meat
- They ate fresh foods
- They kept up strenuous activity throughout their lives
- They liked to do outside work and rose early

"The major characteristic of the diet of longevous people is low total calorie intake throughout life." - Dan Georgakas, *The Methuselah Factors*.

Some of the clinical studies we have of extended human lifespan are documented in the books that are listed in the Bibliography, including *The Methuselah Factors* by Dan Georgakas, *Youth in Old Age* by Alexander Leaf, and *Healthy Aging* by Andrew Weil.

It was only during the last century that nutritionists concluded that the closer an organism (animal or human) comes to its minimal daily food requirements, the longer its lifespan will be. But God was ahead of everyone. He prescribed the quantity of daily food intake, as discussed in the chapter on "The God-given Diet."

Dr. N.W. Walker, whose books are listed in the Bibliography, spent most of his life exploring man's capability to extend life. He lived to be 99 according to the Web, but some sources say 109. His books are referred to several times in this book since they provide much insight into what foods should be eaten for longevity and optimum health.

According to Dr. Walker, the foods that people should eat for longevity are the foods of the raw vegan diet. Raw plant foods are the most conducive of any foods to longevity because they contain an abundance of life force properties and enzymes and do not contain man-made and man-altered ingredients.

Maybe we are only now beginning to understand how to achieve longevity. As discussed in the chapter on "The Dangers of Cooked Foods," enzymes are important life catalysts that are abundant in raw plant foods. Dr. Ann Wigmore, whose books are listed in the Bibliography, believed that enzyme preservation is the secret to longevity.

"Enzymes, apparently, are the key to longevity; they seem to neutralize the basic causes of aging and enable the body to retain its youthful qualities." - Dr. Ann Wigmore, *Be Your Own Doctor.*

A Christian Diet

Christians might ask, "Does being a Christian mean I will live longer than others?" The answer is unabashedly "No." Christians do not live longer than others. In fact, many Christians are called home much sooner than nonbelievers. However, it would seem that Christians are at a "full age" when God takes them home.

Consider the following verse from the Book of Job, "You shall come to the grave at a full age, as a sheaf of grain ripens in its season." - Job 5:26.

Note that it does not say, "at an old age" but "at a full age". All fruits and vegetables do not ripen in the same season. Some are early bloomers and some are late bloomers. And so it is with people. But we, as Christians, will die at a full age. In this, two mercies are shown to us – we will never die too soon, and we will never die too late.

God has put eternity in our hearts (Eccl. 3:11). We were not made for 60 or 70 or 100 years, but for seventy times seven million years. It will take that long to fulfill all of our dreams.

It is our duty to strive for optimum health while we remain in the world of the living. No one knows the day of their death. Happily, we have nothing to do with that date; only God knows its appointed time. But we must be good stewards of our lives and do what is right to promote and sustain our health.

If you seek to extend the term of your existence, then adopt the raw vegan diet, keep physically and mentally active and do not overeat.

The Inevitability of Death

"I shall be satisfied when I awake in Your likeness." - Ps. 17:15.

Except for those who are still alive at the Lord's return (1 Thess. 4:14-17), everyone will pass through the gates of death. Psalm 90 (the prayer of Moses) and Isaiah 40:6-8 describes it as man's inevitable destruction.

Based on the data we have on life expectancy, our lives on earth seem to be limited to 120 years. However, only a few of us will ever live to the great age of 110. Some of us may see a hundred summers, springs, autumns and winters, but most will see no more than seventy of eighty of them.

Everyone shall follow
> As countless have gone before. (Job 21:33)

Death is the end of earthly dreams, friends, pleasures, plans, pains and struggles. We can do much during our days to make the most of things, but we cannot forestall the inevitable.

We know from the Bible that there are three kinds of death: physical, spiritual and eternal. Physical death occurs when the body dies. Spiritual death may occur while we are in this world. A person may be alive physically, but dead spiritually towards God. Those who are spiritually dead do not have the peace, joy and serenity of those who are spiritually alive, who have earnestly asked God, through His Son, for His forgiveness of their sins. Eternal death is separation from God forever, separation from all that is good and beneficial, kind, loving and helpful. Eternal death is said to occur on the Day of Judgement to those who are spiritually dead.

A Christian Diet

The Bible indicates that time as we know it may not exist in the next world. God is beyond time. With Him, a day is as a thousand years and a thousand years is as a day. Our years on earth are not many in the grand scheme of things.

It is God's will that all of His creation must age and die (Isa. 40:6-8; Deut. 32:39). Since God is perfect in all ways and all of His works are perfect, then aging and death must be good things. And we know that all things work together for good to those who love God, to those who are called according to His purpose (Rom. 8:28).

The Bible does not tell us much about the next world. However, it indicates in the Old Testament that when physical death occurs the soul (or spirit) first goes to a place of rest and stays in restful darkness until the Day of Judgment. Many verses indicate this, for example, 1 Kings 2:10, "So David rested with his fathers." The KJV is more specific in that it uses "slept" instead of "rested." Jesus said that the little girl was not dead but sleeping. Both of my parents have died, so they are now sleeping. When I die, I will not meet my parents at first, because I will be sleeping too. When you are dead, you are unconscious like when you are asleep.

Ezekiel 18:4 reveals that the soul is the property of God. Daniel 7:9, and 2 Corinthians 5:10, tell us that on Judgment Day thrones will be set in place and books opened, and that souls will be judged for their actions and their words, for what they did with their time and how they treated others and, in particular, for what they did about God and His Son while in their bodies on earth. Heaven and earth will be witnesses against us. An eternity of life will open for some, and an eternity of torment will open for others. Jesus's words to the repentant thief on the cross indicate that some souls may immediately ascend to heaven (paradise) at death.

Purgatory, which is perhaps a figment of pagan writers, is not mentioned in the Bible.

No one is exempt from the Day of Judgment. All will be judged and sentenced. There are many absolutes in this world -- hot and cold, light and darkness, good and evil, truth and falsehood, love and hate, right and wrong, sacred and profane. Likewise, there is a heaven and an everlasting fire. But only one awaits each of us. The decisions made in life affect our soul's eternal destiny. Some follow the leanings of their spirit as the Master plays on the heart strings, and some do not. Some read the Bible and some do not. Unfortunately for many, an ignorance of God's will on Judgment Day will be of no excuse. As it is known in courts of law, Ignorantia legis neminem excusat, which is Latin for "ignorance of the law excuses no one."

One of our duties as followers of Christ is to contribute to the war against ignorance, replacing, where we can, ignorance with knowledge. God expects enlightened souls to carry the torch for Him here on earth and act as His ambassadors to a lost world.

The mind receives the Word of God through one's sight and hearing, or, in the case of the blind, touch. But it is risky business leaving the words of the Bible to another's interpretation. If practical, everyone should read the Scriptures for themselves, because everyone is expected to know and understand what they says. "How blessed are our ears to hear what God has spoken to us, and to believe what He has written for our learning."

I he Lord is righteous in all his ways
>And holy in all his works. (Ps 145:17)

The Bible is full of examples of the righteousness of God. No one can read the Scriptures without learning about His righteousness.

A Christian Diet

Did we, while in this world, acknowledge Him as Father, and Jesus Christ as His Son? Did we thank Him for giving us the good things that supported and comforted our natural lives? Did we thank Him for the body that we are the caretaker of? Did we thank Him for the air, food, water and health that we enjoy?

"Whosoever shall deny Me before men, him shall I also deny before My Father who is in heaven." - Matt. 10:33.

Many people believe that they are intrinsically accountable to no one but themselves. Pride rules the heart in such cases. But pride separates us from God. It is the worst sin of the Bible because it is rebellion against God. God will not circumvent or countermand a man's gift of free choice. But whatever a man sows that shall he also reap (Gal. 6:7).

To come to God, we must put away our pride long enough to where we do not think so highly of ourselves. While God may not bring on pain and suffering as punishment for our sins (we are more than capable of doing that ourselves in many various ways), He does engineer circumstances in our lives, some for the express purpose of awakening the spirit that lives within us.

A major setback, an extreme disappointment, a serious illness, a loss of something or someone important to us, is often the only thing that will bring us to our knees. It is then, when our hearts are humbled and we turn to Him, that we discover Him. And when we discover Him, we realize that He was there all the time we thought He was not there, and while we were waiting for Him to come to us, He was patiently waiting for us to come to Him. God then enters into a life and gives that life more life (John 10:10).

Without difficult or trying circumstances in our lives, it is hard for us to come to God in faith. It's not easy for a person who's rich in the world's goods and security to have faith in God. As preachers have known, no doubt, from time immemorial, some people have a very hard task to live by faith, and when he or she says, "I trust in God," the probabilities are that they are trusting in their property holdings or savings, and whether it is genuine faith or not is questionable. It is easier to trust God in adversity than in prosperity, for whatever trust there is in adversity is real trust, the genuine article.

Without faith it is impossible to please Him,
For he who comes to God must believe that He is. (Heb. 11:6)

What is the consolation of knowing that we will die? It is that we are on our way home, and that every moment that passes brings us closer to our eternal destination, where we can look forward to knowing Him much better than we do now. We need not fear or worry about the inevitability of death, for heaven will more than compensate for all that we have suffered and lost in this life.

Our Call to the God-given Diet

"And God said, "See, I have given you every herb that yields seed which is on the face of all the earth, and every tree whose fruit yields seed; to you it shall be for food." - Gen. 1:29.

We all learn the importance of taking care of our body sooner or later. While it may not be our main priority, it should be a top priority in our lives. Pope John Paul II said that holiness must be our first priority.

The reluctance of people in this country and in the world to strive to be as healthy as they can be may be due to a number of reasons, but high on the list is the lack of knowledge about foods and nutrition. Also, many of us make a conscious decision every day to continue to satisfy our desires for foods regardless of the health consequences. Others simply do not have the time to pursue better ways of promoting and sustaining their health, which, however, is the same as allowing other things to assume greater priority.

As we learn more about foods and nutrition, and apply the vast storehouse of knowledge that has been gained about how health improvements result from eating natural, untainted foods, we become more aware of what foods do to us and why. An understanding of our own nutritional requirements, and how they are best met by eating whole plant foods, leads us to accepting the truth about Genesis 1:29, and this is confirmed when we experience the phenomenal health improvements that are received on the raw vegan diet.

As discussed throughout this book, when we eat contrary to the laws of nature, a toll is levied on our health that must be paid, and it matters little what belief system we may have since Nature is no respecter of persons. When we break her laws, we can expect to suffer the consequences. But when we abide by them, we can expect to reap the benefits, and that includes optimum health.

Like any other call that is given to us in the Bible, to benefit from the call to the God-given diet (the raw vegan diet), we must respond to it. Either let the truth of the Word of God serve as the motivation to adopt the diet, or let the motivation come from the many health improvements that result from the diet, or let it come from the vastly decreased likelihood of ever getting diseases or other health disorders on the diet. If the motivation is there, the efforts required to make the shift to the diet will follow.

Almost all improvements in life come about from doing new things, even things that may have never been contemplated before. Optimum health results from learning about the nutritional and other needs of the body, and doing the things that meet those needs.

Let the Bible be your guide to optimal health.

The prophet Daniel requested that he and his friends be given vegetables to eat and water to drink for ten days before being compared in appearance to the others who partook of the king's delicacies. At the end of ten days, Daniel and his three friends had features healthier in appearance than the young men who had consumed the king's fare. To me, that says as much about the importance of adopting a whole plant food diet as it does about proper food combining.

Learn about the diet and you will reap the benefits. Do nothing and you will reap the consequences of inaction when action may be just what is needed in your life.

Our call is to the God-given diet (raw vegan diet). As it is said in the Mission Impossible series, "It is your mission, if you choose to accept it."

Transitioning to the God-given Diet

Professor Arnold Ehret and Dr. N. W. Walker, among others, treated critically and hopelessly ill patients by starting them directly on a raw plant food diet, with no intervening transition period, to save their lives and cure their diseases. Complete cures were achieved under the diet. For more details, see the books by these authors that are listed in the Bibliography.

If you or someone you know is currently facing a serious health crisis such as imminent hospitalization or death, then transitioning to the raw vegan diet may not be appropriate. Instead, I would recommend promptly seeking the advice of a qualified homeopathic or naturopathic professional who is familiar with the healing powers of living plant foods, and getting their opinion on starting directly on the raw vegan diet.

Barring such cases, however, I recommend a gradual, but rather swift transition to the raw vegan diet from whatever diet you may be on. The transition is fully explained in this chapter.

This chapter is intended for all who have not attained the diet that consists of eating uncooked whole plant foods exclusively (i.e., the raw vegan diet), and includes those who are currently on the vegetarian and vegan diets. The difference between these diets is explained below.

Raw plant foods promote optimum health and longevity. They give you the zest and energy you always wanted but never could quite obtain. They make you feel good about each and every day of your life. The raw vegan diet literally transforms you into a new person. Other diets cannot do this.

I recommend transitioning to the raw vegan diet by following, in rapid succession, the order of diets listed below. Transition by first becoming a vegetarian, then a vegan and then a raw vegan. The reasons for this are explained in this chapter.

Vegetarian Diet – The vegetarian diet is a diet that consists mostly of plant foods. It minimizes meat and dairy products but can include some fish, and/or some dairy and poultry such as cheese and eggs. The emphasis of the vegetarian diet is on eating mainly plant foods but also cutting back on animal-based foods. Both cooked plant and animal-based foods are allowed on the vegetarian diet.

Vegan Diet – The vegan diet is somewhat like the vegetarian diet but it goes further to exclude all animal-based foods, even fish, cheese and eggs. The vegan diet allows cooked plant foods to be eaten.

Raw Vegan Diet – The raw vegan diet is somewhat like the vegan diet in that it excludes all animal-based foods. But it also excludes all cooked foods, which includes cooked plant foods.

The objective is to attain the raw vegan diet from whatever diet you may currently be on in less than a year. This goal can be achieved even if you are currently on the typical American diet. But it means not wasting anymore time just thinking about switching diets. It means taking the steps necessary to make it happen.

The purpose of the transition period is to learn all that is needed to obtain and maintain the raw vegan diet while suffering the least along the way. Like most changes in life, going through the gears smoothly versus abruptly is easier on the mind and body. You will definitely learn from each of the intermediary diets, but the goal is the raw vegan diet.

It must be emphasized, however, not to dwell in either of the two inferior diets (vegetarian and vegan) for very long. To reach the goal you must keep moving. Plan ahead to go through the two intermediary diets as quickly as possible. The actual time it takes for you to do it will depend on your initiative, persistence and ability to learn new things, but you must keep moving to make it all happen within a year.

You cannot achieve optimal health by making half-hearted attempts at being healthier. This includes remaining on any partially-raw vegan diet like the vegan 80/20 diet (80% raw, 20% cooked) which I was on for a long time. It's like being partially well, which means partially unwell. Actually, the vegan 80/20 diet amounts to being less than 80% well since cooked foods cause toxic buildup in the body tissues which further complicates health. There is no substitute for being 100% healthy. Eating 100% raw plant foods makes you 100% well. Anything short of that does not.

For anyone who is firmly set on eating only raw plant foods starting today, it is possible to jump immediately into the raw vegan diet without a transition period. People have done it. It means quitting harmful foods all at once, which for most people is too big of a change to easily manage, and there are reasons for that.

One of the major obstacles in the way to successfully attaining a whole plant food diet is what I call the curse of "food convenience." Our society is built on fast foods and fast drinks. We need to break away from these things. It requires shifting our focus to healthy foods and drinks, those with health-appeal rather than taste-appeal. It means taking the time required to shop at local food stores for our foods, even though doing so typically takes only minutes more than it does to drive through a fast food place. This may be a major shift in thinking for many people. It's hard to break old habits. However, they were formed by repetition and they can be broken by repeatedly refraining from them.

The foods we are accustomed to eat have strong ties on us. While we may not always be aware of these ties or attractions, they cause cravings. The transition approach helps to deal with these cravings. But whoever has the resolve and willpower to become a raw vegan without transitioning should definitely go for it. If successful, you will be enjoying the rewards of the raw vegan diet that much sooner.

The knowledge acquired about raw plant foods during this period will make you a smarter shopper and assist you in making better food choices, choices based more on health-appeal than taste-appeal.

An important concept to include in one's thinking about foods is that they are a source of medicine as well as nourishment. When this concept is internalized, great strides in health are possible.

"Let food be thy medicine and medicine be thy food." - Hippocrates.

THINGS TO LEARN DURING THE TRANSITION PERIOD

• The difference between ripe and un-ripe produce.

• Shelf and refrigerator life of most fruits and vegetables.

• What fruits and vegetables can be frozen and not frozen.

- How to read food labels, and what ingredients to avoid.

- The dangers of pesticides.

- The benefits of organic foods.

- The food combination laws.

- What detoxification is, and how to speed up the process.

- How to perform colonics and enemas.

You will learn many of these things by reading this book.

The ancient Roman caution, "Caveat Emptor" ("Let the Buyer Beware"), carries the same weight and significance now as it did in the days of the Roman Empire. It is our responsibility to avoid foods and ingredients that are harmful to us. During the transition period, you will learn to analyze the food labels and understand what they mean.

No matter where you are on the raw vegan diet journey, you can improve your health today simply by quitting one or two harmful foods or ingredients and replacing them with healthier choices. Then, after several weeks, declare victory and move on to quit another food or ingredient, replacing it with a healthier choice. In this way, you progress to the raw vegan diet.

Eliminating all meat and dairy products, refined sugar and refined salt from your diet is a huge step in the right direction. It will be your first goal if you are not already there. It means stop eating fast foods, including energy drinks, sodas and colas, most restaurant foods and refined and processed foods. In the place of meat and dairy products, eat raw fruits, vegetables and leafy greens, and get used to them. Then expand your food selections to include different varieties than those you are already used to. Start using natural, unrefined sea salt (see the chapter on "The Good and Bad About Salt.")

During the transition period, some cooked foods may be eaten. The reason for this is explained below. Remember, however, that the goal is to quit eating cooked foods. Also, my recommendation is to stop eating all starchy foods. Previous chapters of this book have described the dangers of consuming these foods.

Get to where you are eating at least one meal a day of only raw fruit and maybe also greens (e.g., a green smoothie for breakfast). Raw fruits counteract many of the harmful effects of a mixed diet, that is, a cooked food and raw food diet. Eating more raw fruit (fresh or sun-dried) during the transition period will be of benefit to the cells of the body and will enhance the self-cleansing process.

It is during the transition period that the food combination laws are learned. Plan on making mistakes; it's part of any learning experience.

THINGS NEEDED FOR THE RAW VEGAN DIET

• Cutting boards of different sizes

• Knives

• Knife sharpening stone

• Blender

• Lemon/lime squeezer

- Glass or plastic jars with tops (for green smoothies on the go)

If you have never sharpened a knife on a stone, then it's time to learn. A dull knife in the kitchen makes many things more difficult.

I use a reconditioned Vitamix blender and have never had a problem with it. It's probably the only blender I will ever need. Before the Vitamix, I went through several retail store blenders, burning out the motors. Vitamix claims you really have to push the blender to warm foods above 115 degrees F, and I have yet to use it on its maximum speed. The Vitamix container is BPA-free plastic, versus glass, which makes it light weight and easy to clean.

The best lemon/lime squeezer, in my opinion, is a stainless steel, hand-held model. It takes very little pressure to squeeze out the juice of a lemon or lime or other citrus fruit.

Detoxification

Detoxification is the process by which the body auto-cleanses itself of toxic wastes. The body is always trying to purge itself of toxins, but certain foods hinder the process. Detoxification really takes off when raw plant foods are consumed exclusively. If you are on an ordinary diet, the detoxification process is, for all practical purposes, ineffectual because ordinary diets cause toxic wastes to build up to the extent where thorough detoxification is not possible. The detoxification process is also known as self-purification or self-cleansing.

Detoxification is the healthy ridding of the body of its accumulated toxins. The process typically causes more frequent defecations and urinations, and maybe some diarrhea. These things are normal and last only during the cleansing process.

Detoxification is how the body heals and rejuvenates itself. Whole plant foods give the body what it needs for self-cleansing and provide it with the best raw materials for cellular reconstruction. Detoxification is the rite of passage everyone must go through to become genuinely healthy. Internal cleansing is required before rejuvenation and optimum health can be achieved.

Toxins accumulate in the organs and tissues of the body from eating animal-based foods, cooked and starchy foods and refined and processed foods. They also accumulate when inorganic multivitamin/mineral supplements are taken, for reasons that have already been discussed. The body also gets toxins from the environment, e.g., from exhaust fumes, municipal drinking water, etc.

When the body contains many poisons and is daily given more of them through the foods that are eaten, ill-health reigns. When the body is cleansed of its toxins and is daily given living plant foods, health reigns.

Raw plant foods possess the highest level of nutrients found in any food, and bestow numerous health benefits, some of which are yet to be discussed in this book. An abundance of vitality is available to anyone who adopts the raw vegan diet. When toxins are removed from the body through the self-cleansing process that is enhanced by eating raw plant foods, you feel great.

What is known as "toxic overload" may occur when the detoxification/self-cleansing process is ramped into high gear by a sudden shift to an all whole plant food diet.

The sudden shift causes an abundance of toxins to be released into the bloodstream all at once, and, as confirmed by many raw food eaters and nutritional experts, this may cause flu or disease like symptoms to occur creating discomfort and malaise. People have gotten seriously ill from transitioning too quickly to the raw vegan diet. This is why a gradual transition to the raw vegan diet is recommended. The purpose of eating some cooked foods during the transition period is to slow down the detoxification process in order to avoid toxic overload.

Living plant foods are so powerful that they immediately start cleansing the body of its poisons. Their life force actions on the body drive out toxic wastes into the bloodstream for their elimination through the normal elimination organs of the body (including the skin). The powers of living plant foods are clearly evidenced by the signs the body gives when it detoxifies itself on these foods.

David Wolfe in his book, *The Sunfood Diet Success System*, states that detoxification stops when cooked food is eaten. The dangers associated with cooked foods, why they are detrimental to human health, are described in the chapter on "The Dangers of Cooked Foods."

Wastes released into the system from eating a whole plant food diet initially make you feel unhealthy, and during the self-cleansing process you may experience some signs of ill-health. But that is natural and normal. It is caused by the toxins within the tissues and organs of the body being released into the bloodstream. Feelings of fatigue, dizziness, and the signs cited below may be experienced until the "house cleaning" is completed. But when the toxins are eliminated, the feeling of true health is experienced.

The possible ill effects of detoxification should not in any way dissuade the reader from proceeding with a whole plant food diet, since it is the way to true health. They are provided so that you will not be surprised by them when you undergo detoxification.

Normal signs of detoxification include: frequent urinations and/or bowel movements, diarrhea, headaches, runny nose, colds, expectoration, loss of energy, feelings of melancholy, needing more sleep, etc., all indications that the body is purging itself of toxins. Additional signs of detoxification are found in Robert Morse's book, *The Detox Miracle Sourcebook*.

We need to take detoxification into stride when we start eating raw plant foods exclusively. Continue through the healing process trusting that the body is gaining health by what it is doing. Know that drugs that block these symptoms also block the healing process.

The transient discomforts of detoxification cause some people to quit a whole plant food diet like the raw vegan diet before the benefits are obtained because they do not understand the detoxification process. But those who stick with the process experience the tremendous boost in vitality that follows self-cleansing, when the accumulated poisons are removed from the system.

"There is only one true healing modality – detoxification. It will bring the body's chemistry back into homeostasis (balance) and remove the toxic metals, elements and substances that don't belong there." - Robert Morse, N.D., *The Detox Miracle Sourcebook*.

Those who have never experienced detoxification cannot know what it is like. You can read about it in books, like this one, and in articles on the Web, but unless you have personally gone through it you will never know what it is like.

"A pure raw plant diet assists the body's cleansing efforts in the most natural way by eliminating any toxicity from entering the system and by simultaneously moving toxicity through the lymph and blood and out the body through the eliminating organs (the bowels, kidneys, liver, skin, sinuses and lungs). A purification of the diet enforces a self-healing and radical whole-body rejuvenation." - David Wolfe, *The Sunfood Diet Success System.*

In my opinion, the chief importance of detoxification is to relieve the body of the burden of all forms of constipation, to peel away the coating of paste-like plaque that has formed on the walls of the intestines after years of eating the wrong foods, foods that are detrimental to health (see the chapter on "The Dangers of Starchy Foods").

One of the things I learned during my first year on the raw vegan diet that was not covered in the books listed in the Bibliography, was that improper, or bad, food combinations can cause not only stomachache, headache, heartburn, and flatulence, but also constipation.

Colonics and Enemas

"Death begins in the colon." - Elie Metchnikoff.

Nutritional experts contend that many of the problems we are now facing, including age-related health disorders, are due to the condition of our colons. But they go further and tell us that many, if not most, diseases of humankind originate in the colon. This incredible assertion is explained in the books by Arnold Ehret, Dr. Ann Wigmore and Dr. N. W. Walker that are listed in the Bibliography, and is supported by other nutritional experts.

Hippocrates said, "All disease begins in the gut."

"Your constitutional encumbrances throughout the entire system are the source of every disease; the greatest and most harmful source of lowered vitality, imperfect health, lack of strength and endurance and any and all imperfect conditions. All have their source in the colon, never perfectly emptied since your birth." - Arnold Ehret, *The Mucusless Diet Healing System*.

What if we acted on this information? If there is a direct link between the diseases of humankind and the condition of the colon, shouldn't we do whatever is possible to eliminate toxic waste buildup and the plate-out of the plaque in the colon? Of course we should, and each of us can.

Colonics and enemas help to remove the plaque-like deposits in our colons and release and move toxins out of our systems. In this way, they accelerate the self-cleansing and healing process of the body. Nutritional experts Arnold Ehret, Dr. Norman Walker and others consider colonics and enemas either highly advantageous or absolutely necessary for healing chronic diseases.

If you have never had a colonic or enema, you are not alone. Most people have never had them, and many have never even heard of them. However, as we journey to optimum health we become more and more our own doctors. The transition to the raw vegan diet is the time to learn what these procedures are and how to perform them.

Colonics (also known as colon irrigations or colon hydrotherapy), are procedures performed in the privacy of a personal suite at a local colonic establishment. They help clean out the toxins and wastes accumulated in the colon.

Colonic establishments are located in most cities. The average cost for a colonic irrigation (or hydrotherapy) ranges $60-$100 and you can purchase multiple sessions to save money. I have done the colon hydrotherapy several times. The machine is self-operated and easy to use. You can control it at your own pace for as long as you want. For me, that was about 30 minutes. I decided on the colonics after I read the books by Dr. N.W. Walker in the Bibliography, and particularly his book, *Become Younger.*

A less expensive way to help the detoxification process is to perform enemas at home. Enema kits are available at most retail stores (Wal-Mart, drug stores, etc.). Each kit has a number of small plastic bottles that contain a saline solution. The procedure is to lie down, turn on one side and insert the tip of the bottle and squeeze the bottle. I discovered that better results are obtained by replacing half of the saline solution with freshly-squeezed lemon juice, and using 2 bottles at a time instead of one.

Other types of enema kits are available, such as the travel-bag variety which consists of a long plastic tube and a plastic bag that can be hung from a door knob.

Doing enemas is a good, positive change to make in your life. It is a learning experience that many would much rather avoid, but again, you are becoming more and more your own doctor as you continue on the raw vegan journey.

If you have less than three bowel movements a day then you should be doing colonics and/or enemas on a more frequent basis than once a month. Otherwise, once a month is recommended.

Colonics and enemas are not coffee-table topics for discussion. They are real-world procedures that need to be understood if anyone is serious about achieving optimum health.

For a more thorough discussion of the need for colonics and enemas, see the books by Arnold Ehret and N.W. Walker in the Bibliography.

Remember, if optimum health and longevity required no knowledge or effort or discernment whatsoever on the part of the individual, then they would be easy to come by and everyone would have them. If optimum health could be sold as a magic pill or silver bullet, anyone could easily become healthy without the slightest effort, and this book would not be written. But all things are given to us at the price of labor.

"The "basement" of the human "temple" is the reservoir from which every symptom of disease and weakness is supplied in all its manifestations." - Arnold Ehret, *The Mucusless Diet Healing System*.

If you actively incorporate the information contained in this chapter into your life, you will be doing your health a great service, and perhaps more than you may realize.

Fasting

I consider fasting to be instrumental to the attainment of optimum health, even if it means just skipping a meal occasionally or practicing the no-breakfast plan, which is further discussed in the chapter on "Vitality."

The history of fasting, its many benefits to human health were covered in the chapter on "The Importance of Fasting." As explained therein, fasting acts so powerfully on the body that many diseases can be completely cured through its practice alone. For this reason, I highly recommend that some type of fasting be regularly practiced if the aim is to achieve and maintain optimum health.

If fasting can cure almost all human diseases, what does that tell us about how diseases and other health disorders originate? It clearly indicates that the principle cause of disease lies in the foods that are eaten, and it implicates many of our ailments with improper diet. This, of course, is what nutritionists have been telling us for years.

Fasting is so significant to the attainment of genuine health that if the reader gets nothing out of this book but the importance of fasting, then the book will have served its purpose, because fasting signifies, and in the practice of fasting is found, almost all of the health principles that are elucidated in this book.

As explained in this chapter on transitioning to the raw vegan diet, many new things need to be learned on the journey to optimum health. Foremost among them are detoxification, colonics, enemas and fasting.

If you do not know how to do the things described in this chapter, but you seriously want to have the best of health, then you should learn how to do them. It is all part of the adventure.

"Our joy, our happiness is in growing." - Alfred Armand Montapert.

Why Other Diets Cannot Deliver Vibrant Health

The two diets that come closest to the raw vegan diet (God-given diet) are the vegetarian and vegan diets. Both were described in the previous chapter. There is no need to discuss other diets, including the many fad diets that come out each year (e.g., the various high-protein, high-fat and low-carb diets) since animal products and cooked foods, which are part of these diets, are harmful to the body, as maintained by many noted nutritionists and as explained in this book.

Both the vegetarian and vegan diets restrict, or avoid, animal-based foods, which is to their credit. However, both allow cooked foods to be eaten, which is to their detriment, since cooked foods are harmful to human health.

The cooking of foods at home and in restaurants, and in the food factories that manufacture canned, bottled and jarred foods, reduces the food value of the foods by altering their chemical properties and destroying important food components, such as enzymes and nutrients, including vitamins and antioxidants.

If food is browned by heat treatment, such as by broiling, baking or deep frying, dangerous chemicals are created, such as advanced glycation end-products (AGEs), which have been known to cause diabetes and heart disease as discussed in the chapter on "The Dangers of Cooked Foods."

Almost every kind of food that comes in a sealed package (bag, box, can, jar, bottle, etc.) has been refined and processed, meaning, among other things, that it has been heat-treated. The enzymes in the foods have been destroyed by heat, and superfluous and harmful substances have been added as discussed previously in this book. Refined and processed foods are responsible for a large number of health disorders, ranging from headaches to the top 10 leading causes of diseases in this country, and most diets permit these foods to be eaten.

Nothing that man can do to foods, such as high temperature heat treatment, the addition of preservatives, artificial colors and sweeteners, antibiotics (in animal products), and other refined and/or man-made ingredients, can improve the food value of foods over their living food counterparts. To think that it can is ludicrous, since anything done by man to foods (other than necessary harvesting or shipping) alters or adulterates the foods in some way.

As explained in the chapter on "The Foods We Should Eat and Why," the foods that we should eat are not the refined and processed man-made foods that many of us grew up on, including the many fast foods and meat and dairy products that are commonly consumed, but the foods that God made specifically for us, foods that we are biologically suited for: raw plant foods.

The body's ability to fight illnesses is determined by the health of the immune system. Certain diseases, including cancer, repress the immune system and allow increased attacks by unfriendly microbes, including the smallest of microbes, the viruses. Nutritionists tell us that the best way to improve the health of the immune system is to eat plenty of whole plant foods.

The raw vegan diet enables us to heal ourselves of diseases and prevent them from taking root in the body, all due to the cleansing and rejuvenating actions that raw plant foods have on us. They enable us to feel better about every day of our lives and be more productive at whatever we do. They eliminate fatigue and enable us to jump-start our lives in profound and singular ways that are not possible with other diets.

As discussed in the chapter on "Antioxidants," the raw vegan diet is the best assurance anyone can have of getting the antioxidants that are needed for health.

Raw plant foods lower body mass index (BMI), meaning body fat, which results in decreased risks of high blood pressure, elevated serum cholesterol, cardiovascular disease, type 2 diabetes and cancers. A plant-based diet is the only diet that has been shown to reverse diseases. Examples are ischemic heart disease (i.e., insufficient blood supply) and type 2 diabetes. The research conducted by Dr. Caldwell Esselstyn, Jr. on how raw plant foods prevent and reverse heart disease Is well known and was described in the chapter on "The Foods We Should Eat and Why."

The results of many dietary studies, some of which are backed by the latest scientific understanding about foods and nutrition, and the wealth of knowledge that is now available that indisputably links improper diet with diseases and other health issues, all point to the importance of eating a whole plant food diet, such as the raw vegan diet, for promoting and sustaining optimum health.

Natural cures have one thing in common, they aim at correcting the underlying causes of health disorders instead of suppressing the symptoms.

Before educating myself about foods and nutrition, I naively believed that food was merely something to satisfy my hunger pangs and reward my taste buds. When I became convinced that a whole plant food diet was the right kind of diet for my health, I had to unlearn about as much as I had previously learned about foods. I slowly but steadily transitioned to a vegetarian diet, then to a vegan diet, before adopting the raw vegan diet.

In the process, I began to view foods as what they really are: life-givers or life-takers. Foods and dietary practices, such as proper food combining, are either conducive to health or injurious to it. I've aged since my quest for the answers began, but I'm now more convinced than ever that a whole plant food diet is the best diet for health.

While I was on the vegan diet, my health stalled. It just stopped improving. And when health stops improving, it typically starts to decline. I didn't know why my health wasn't improving, but I continued to search for the answers. The books I read talked a lot about the importance of eating raw (uncooked) plant foods for energy and disease prevention. Slowly, this information began to sink in. When I became convinced of the dangers of eating cooked foods, I quit cooked foods and became a raw vegan. That was one of the best decisions I ever made.

Because of the raw vegan diet, I no longer consider myself an unsuspecting, gullible food shopper, believing everything the free enterprise system wants me to believe about what is best for my health, because I now know what is best for my health. Because of raw plant foods, I am no longer attracted to, or interested in, fast foods or drinks.

When on the vegetarian and vegan diets, prior to the raw vegan diet, I suffered from various health issues, including constipation, stomachaches, headaches, hemorrhoids, psoriasis and other skin conditions, general fatigue, flatulence (excessive gas), broken sleeps and nightmares. These conditions are so prevalent in our society that they are considered normal conditions of modern life.

But the only thing normal about them is that they are normal signs of ill-health.

In response to these "normal" conditions, entire industries have been created to produce prescription drugs to help people deal with them. Despite the availability of these drugs, I did my best to understand why, from a science of nutrition point of view, I was suffering from my conditions and what steps to take to correct them. I read all I could about each of my conditions. As it turned out, the conditions I had served as the catalyst I needed to change my diet to the raw vegan diet.

It was only after adopting the raw vegan diet that my health really improved. After being on the diet for only a short time, many of the ill-health conditions I had disappeared, and I found myself for the first time in years with a surplus of energy. Just as significantly, my health continues to improve on the diet.

Moreover, many of the foods that are commonly consumed create toxicity or acidity in the body, conditions that are known to be precursors of sickness and disease, and some foods clog up the system causing constipation, which is a known precursor of disease.

The dangers of GMO foods were described in the chapter on "GMO Crops." Upwards of 75% of the refined and processed foods on supermarket shelves contain GMO products. GMO sweet corn and sugar beets are widely used in refined and processed foods as "sugar" or high-fructose corn syrup (HFCS). GMO soybeans are widely used as soy in many refined and processed foods. Soy is found in almost all baked goods and imitation dairy products, and also in alternative meat products such as veggie burgers. Soy derivatives include hydrolyzed plant protein (HPP), hydrolyzed soy protein (HSP) and/or hydrolyzed vegetable protein (HVP), which are added to a wide range of refined and processed foods, including soda, chips, salad dressings and soups.

Dr. J. C. Jarvis, in his book, *Arthritis & Folk Medicine*, emphasizes the importance of diet when taking cures for diseases, such as arthritis. He calls for eliminating acid-producing foods like those found in ordinary diets, including the vegetarian and vegan diets.

"Biologic food selection is followed every day. This removes wheat foods, wheat cereals, white sugar, citrus fruits and their juices, and muscle meats like beef, lamb, and pork from the daily food intake." - Dr. D. C. Jarvis, *Arthritis & Folk Medicine*.

Raw plant foods provide us with numerous health benefits, some of which are yet to be described in this book. An abundance of vitality is available to anyone who adopts the raw vegan diet. When the toxins are removed by the body's self-cleansing process which is enhanced by eating raw plant foods, you feel great.

The foods that are best for us are foods that have their life-giving properties intact, that enable the body to withstand the onslaught of diseases, that provide the energy needed for an active and productive life and that promote and sustain optimum health. Nutritional experts agree that a whole plant food diet, such as the raw vegan diet, minimizes bodily toxicity and acidity and rids the body of its toxins better than any other diet.

The Essene Gospel of Peace

"You will show me the path of life." - Ps. 16:11.

Not many people are aware of the remarkable little book, *The Essene Gospel of Peace, Book One.* It was first translated in the 1920s by Edmond Szekely from the original Aramaic manuscript he found in the Secret Archives of the Vatican, and also from the original Hebrew text he found in the Scriptorium of the Benedictine Monastery of Monte Cassino.

First published in 1928, it is the result of much scholarship, patience and unerring intuition on Szekely's part. His discovery of the manuscripts is documented in the book, *The Discovery of the Essene Gospel of Peace*, published in 1937.

Szekely believed that the manuscripts he used for the book proved that the Essenes were vegetarians, and that vegetarianism was prescribed by Jesus.

Despite the book's title, it does not discuss the Essenes, who were a sect of the Jews living in the desert (near where the Dead Sea Scrolls were discovered) at the time when Jesus walked the earth. Also, the book does not indicate that Jesus was a member of the Essenes, or that he lived among them, as some have since assumed. But the principal character of the book is Jesus.

The book is a rendering of teachings of Jesus about foods and nutrition. It describes what he purported said to his disciples about how foods should be eaten (i.e., combined), what foods are best for us to eat, and how diseases are cured through proper diet and fasting. Basically, it says is that we should eat raw plant foods, abstain from all meat and cooked foods, take frequent enemas to cleanse the colon, and fast. The diet is very similar to that of Genesis 1:29.

The book confirms what many nutritionists have stressed for years about how cooked foods destroy health and weaken the body's capacity to ward off diseases, and about the health benefits of raw plant foods and the importance of fasting in healing diseases. The book has clarified much for me about how optimum health is attainable through proper diet and fasting.

I believe that Jesus is speaking to us from its pages. One of the reasons I believe it is that 'His ways are higher than our ways, and His thoughts than our thoughts' (Isaiah 55:8). Another reason is, "My sheep hear My voice, and I know them, and they follow Me." (John 10:27). The words of Jesus in Szekely's book sound like the words of Jesus in the Bible.

John said in his gospel, "And there are also many other things that Jesus did, which if they were written one by one, I suppose that even the world itself could not contain the books that would be written." I have always believed that.

The book seems to fill-in information about Jesus' teachings on diet that we do not have from the Scriptures, including what foods we should eat and why, how Mother Nature and her angels assist us in health, and the importance of fasting in curing diseases.

The Bible gives us much on the subject of moral conduct, but does not tell us a lot about foods and nutrition. For example, it does not elaborate or explain to any length why we should eat only seed-bearing plants, or how our foods should be eaten. For the first, it just tells us we are to do so, and for the second, it leaves it up to us. Also, in my opinion, it does not provide much detail about how to cure our diseases, and I base this conclusion on reading The Essene Gospel of Peace, which tells us how to cure diseases.

The main passages of the Bible that describe what foods we should eat are those found in Genesis 1, Genesis 9, Leviticus 11, and Deuteronomy 14. In Leviticus 11 and Deuteronomy 14, we have the clean and unclean animal passages. For example, in Leviticus 1:2, God said, "These are the living things that you may eat among all the animals that are on the earth..." The words, "may eat," indicate permission rather than commandment. The words are used in both Leviticus 11 and Deuteronomy 14.

Commandments in the Bible typically use the word "shall", particularly in the earlier translations of the Bible. The two passages about foods that contain "shall" are Genesis1:29 and Genesis 9:3. Genesis 1:29 reads, "And God said, "See, I have given you every herb that yields seed which is on the face of all the earth, and every tree whose fruit yields seed; to you it shall be for food." Genesis 9:3 reads, "Every moving thing that lives shall be food for you. I have given you all things, even as the green herbs."

Genesis 1:29 is clear. However, discussion is necessary regarding Genesis 9:3. In Genesis 9:3, other foods in addition to the seed-bearing plants of Genesis 1:29 were given to man to eat after the Flood. Let's explore this further and see what we may conclude.

God made man without sin and gave him a diet in that condition. It is apparent that after the Fall, however, man learned to eat foods that were inconsistent with the God-given diet. For example, it is only after the Fall that the Bible indicates foods were prepared by fire.

God permitted the eating of animal foods after the Flood but not before. Some believe it was for survival purposes, since there appears to have been a rapid cooldown of the world after the Flood, as evidenced by the frozen woolly mammoths found in Siberia and the ice age that occurred about that time. It rained so much during the Flood that when God sent the winds that dried up the waters, it cooled down the earth in a way similar to the way temperatures drop after a rain, but much more so due to the amount of water involved and the great amount of evaporation that took place. And don't forget that the energy required to change water from a liquid to a gas (vapor) is a lot of heat energy, as we know from boiling water. The energy in this case came from the winds and the heat that was removed from the earth and atmosphere during the evaporation of the Flood waters, the extensive evaporation that caused a rapid deep freezing of the earth. Man needed animal foods to survive the aftermath of the cataclysm.

The guiding precepts for my life, including what my diet should be, have for some time been those found in the Bible, even though some of them may not be completely or thoroughly explained to my satisfaction.

Francis A. Shaeffer states in his book *Escape from Reason*:

"It is an important principle to remember, in the contemporary interest in communication and in language study, that the biblical presentation is that, though we do not have exhaustive truth, we have from the Bible what I term true truth. In this way we know true truth about God, true truth about man, and something truly about nature. Thus, on the basis of the Scriptures, while we do not have exhaustive knowledge, we have true and unified knowledge."

As explained by Jesus in the New Testament, such as in Matt. 19:7-8, and Matt. 5:21 through the end of the chapter, the instruction that was given to the children of Israel in the desert during their 40 years of disbelief was not necessarily what God originally intended for them to receive, but was other instruction that they could more easily follow. It is apparent from Jesus's statements that the advice God originally gave the children of Israel was ignored, or it was tried and rejected by them as being too difficult to obey. Stephen tells us much the same in Acts 7:39. Therefore, much of the instruction Moses ended up giving them was instruction that they could more easily follow, which was still a giant step above what they were accustomed to in Egypt, with every man doing what was right in his own eyes.

Proper diet, a knowledge of fasting and how to cure diseases are not necessary for salvation, which is the message of the Bible, but they are important for health and well-being, and for developing a heightened sense of spirituality.

We do not know what Jesus ate on a daily basis. But it is apparent that meager fare was a complete meal for Him. The Bible indicates that He must have been thin because He fasted often to heal the sick. He could not carry His cross to the outskirts of the city, although the other two condemned men apparently had no problem carrying theirs after they, too, had been scourged. We know that all three were scourged because scourging was a legal preliminary to every Roman execution.

I believe *The Essene Gospel of Peace* was given to us to help understand more about foods and nutrition and how diseases may be healed through proper diet and fasting. The many quotations from the book that are included in this book attest to this belief. No other book that I am aware of complements the teachings of the Bible regarding foods and nutrition and how to heal the sick as well as *The Essene Gospel of Peace.*

Part of the duty we have to ourselves, and part of our duty as stewards of everything that God has placed under our control, is to understand how we should live out our lives. As emphasized in this book, a knowledge of foods and nutrition is crucial to healthy living and good stewardship.

Read *The Essene Gospel of Peace* for yourself, and see if it doesn't strike a chord of truth in you about what we should eat and how diseases may be cured.

We are well-pleasing to God whenever we can solve our own problems by using what He has given us, our minds and abilities, our desire to learn new things, our resolve and our faith.

"But whoever keeps His word, truly the love of God is perfected in him. By this we know that we are in Him. He who says he abides in Him ought himself also to walk just as He walked." - 1 John 2:5-6.

Vitality

"It is not that someone else is preventing you from living happily; you yourself do not know what you want. Rather than admit this, you pretend that someone is keeping you from exercising your liberty. Who is this? It is you yourself." - Thomas Merton, *New Seeds of Contemplation.*

Vitality is defined as the state of being strong and active. It is said to be the power that runs the human machine. It is physical and mental vigor. Vitality is what all of us want more of, what others expect more of us, and what everyone over 65 strives to obtain.

We are vital organisms and function through vital processes, many of which are operating without our awareness, such as homeostasis and cellular reconstruction. Lasting vitality, the kind that doesn't leave you but stays with you, is directly related to the internal cleanliness of the body. If your body has been cleansed of its toxins and wastes, you wake up feeling exuberant instead of fatigued. It's the secret of the ancients, and it is now available to us.

As we age, most of us view every day as a struggle. But it doesn't have to be that way. When you have gone through detoxification on the raw vegan diet, you can enjoy a great deal of vitality that others do not have, which enables you to turn many of your struggles into solutions.

"It has been my experience that once the body has been thoroughly cleansed and has become accustomed to such a regime for several months or years, the individual becomes indefatigable, with an almost inexhaustible supply of energy, vigor and vitality, as well as an astonishing amount of strength and endurance." - Dr. Norman W. Walker, *The Vegetarian Guide to Diet and Salad.*

As discussed previously, proper eating habits help determine vitality, since every ounce of food that passes through the body that is not actually needed taxes the body's vital powers, and is a waste of vital energy.

It has been proposed by some nutritionists, including Edward Hooker Dewey, Hereward Carrington and Wallace D. Wattles (their books are listed in the Bibliography), that vitality is not manufactured by the body from foods that we eat, but, rather, flows into us from the great Eternal Source (presumedly God) when we are asleep. This is called the "vitality theory."

The vitality theory may, at first, sound strange, even unbelievable, but after reading this chapter you will see that there is a lot of truth in it.

The theory is based on the assertion that foods do not really energize us at all, but act only as stimulants. This is contrary to what is commonly believed by almost everyone, including our doctors -- that foods are required for the body to produce and sustain energy and health.

Sick and diseased patients, whether in or out of hospital, are encouraged by their doctors to take nourishment to get well (and in hospitals patients eat the food from hospital kitchens!). This long-held and firmly entrenched belief has been indolibly engraved upon our minds. However, as discussed in the chapter on "The Importance of Fasting," clinical studies conducted on fasting indicate that when sick we should eat nothing.

The vitality theory contends that foods do not energize us, but only provide the raw materials for the rebuilding of the body's cells. The more physically active we are, the more food we need for cellular reconstruction. The theory postulates that we do not get energy from foods, but that it comes to us from the Eternal Source. Furthermore, it argues that our receptivity to this energy is increased when the body is in a healthy condition. When we maintain the body in a healthy condition by eating foods that promote and sustain health, that is, whole plant foods, this receptivity is heightened.

There is something remarkable and even revolutionary about the vitality theory. It seems to fit in well with the mystery of life as we know it, and our common conception of God being the infinite source of all things.

The idea that energy flows into the sleeping brain from an outside source rather than being supplied by the foods that we eat would be easy to refute if there were no truth in it. It could easily be refuted by performing a simple exercise or experiment. All that would be necessary would be for us to eat a meal and show that a full stomach increases vitality.

However, we know that meals tax our energies, and that digestion is, perhaps as it is claimed, the greatest energy requirement of the body. More often than not after eating a meal, we feel sluggish or tire easily because of the internal energy being expended.

When I fasted for 5 days, the work that I was doing was not hindered in the slightest; I remained fully productive at work all during the fast.

In addition, if food were all that were needed for vitality, then we would never need to rest or sleep, but would be able to keep on eating and working indefinitely. However, we know that this is not true. No matter how much food we may consume during the day, at the end of the day we feel exhausted. Our days are, in fact, ruined by lack of vitality whenever we are deprived of sufficient sleep.

In addition, during severe sickness, Nature takes away our appetite for food. This is consistent with the vitality theory since during sickness no internal power should be spared while the body is fighting the sickness, and it takes power to run the stomach to digest food.

All living things sleep -- humans, animals, fish, reptiles, insects, even plants. All require periods of slumber. Ever wonder why all lifeforms sleep? According to the Web at the time of this writing, scientists do not know why all creatures sleep. According to the vitality theory, it's because life needs to be recharged with the vital energy that comes from above.

"Life is an energy which is stored in the brain during sleep. If we understand that material food plays no part in the generation of that energy, and govern our appetites accordingly, we shall have perfect health." - Wallace D. Wattles, *Health Through New Thought and Fasting.*

The theory also seems to fit in well with the fact that raw plant foods enhance spirituality, since they, and especially fruits, are very cleansing to the body. Also, it helps to explain why fasting enhances spirituality since food is withheld during fasting which promotes internal cleansing.

Food, then, according to the vitality theory, is not the primary source of physical power. Rather, it is to the body what raw materials are to the builder. Food, in this view, has two main functions. It is required for the replacement of the body's cells, and for enhancing the receptivity of the brain to the vital force that comes to us from the Infinite while we sleep. While foods do have caloric energy, meals tax our energies. We need sleep to recharge the energy reserves of the body.

The old saying that cleanliness is next to godliness takes on a new meaning in connection with the vitality theory.

Many nutritionists believe in the vitality theory. They argue that all we have to do to be good receivers of this energy is to keep the body clean and free of disease.

Scientists know that if the facts do not support a theory, then the theory must be readjusted, or discarded, to fit the facts. But in this case, many facts, as indicated above, support the theory.
Based on my research of relevant material from books and the Web at the time of this writing, there seems to be very little, if any, clinical evidence to support the vitality theory, that vitality comes from an outside source of power. Some may argue that the power is transmitted in ways that we cannot yet detect. Although this is reasonable, it is mere speculation.

A few results have appeared in brain research that indicate there is a connection between sleep and vitality, but none I am aware of that support the "transmission of power" hypothesis of the vitality theory.

Doctors at the Department of Human Health Sciences, Kyoto University Graduate School of Medicine, in Japan, found that the quality of sleep a person gets directly affects a person's vitality. But this is only to be expected, since a lack of sleep adversely affects vitality.

Several years ago, Dr. Maiken Nedergaard, a professor of neurosurgery and co-director of the Center for Translational Neuromedicine at the University of Rochester Medical Center, discovered an important nervous system mechanism in the brain that prevents waste products from building up in the brain. She called it the "glymphatic system." The glymphatic system flushes any "debris" from the brain to the liver where it is eliminated.

According to the NIH (National Institutes of Health) Record of April 2015, Dr. Nedergaard reviewed a number of theories about what makes sleep a biological imperative, including its benefits to memory, the immune system and the preservation of human energy. She believes that sleep plays an important role in regulating the glymphatic system. Advanced imaging technology such as two-photon microscopy was used to examine the brains of live mice. The experiments compared the brains of mice that were awake, asleep and under anesthesia, to see if there was any difference in the way the glymphatic system worked to flush out the wastes from the brain. They found that during sleep, the glymphatic system was 10 times more active than when the mice were awake.

We always knew that sleep was good for us. Dr. Nedergaard's research indicates that there may be a connection between the preservation of human energy and the brain being cleansed of its waste products during sleep. But again, this evidence is far from supporting certain aspects of the vitality theory.

In any event, there is more. The new physiology expounded in this chapter recommends skipping breakfast entirely. One of the first to propose it as a means to a healthier and more vibrant life was Edward Hooker Dewey. He called it the "No-Breakfast Plan" in his book, *The No-Breakfast Plan and the Fasting Cure*.

The NB plan makes sense. According to Harvey Diamond (two of his books are listed in the Bibliography), the body's elimination cycle extends from the time we go to sleep at night until noon the following day. It is during this time that the body's self-cleansing process focuses on eliminating waste products from the system. For the cycle to be truly effective, no food should be eaten during this time. That makes perfect sense to me.

I've adopted the no-breakfast plan in my daily regimen. and find that breakfast is not needed at all for energy and stamina. The energy levels I have without breakfast are higher than when I ate breakfast. During this time of no nourishment, I work out strenuously at the gym and do my office work. I'm never lacking in energy during this time or at any other time for that matter. I break the fast by eating raw fruit. Later in the mornings I eat a mixed raw vegetable salad. Initially, I had gone until noon without eating, which I found was just too long a period of being without food for me.

People eat breakfast mostly out of habit. As discussed in the chapter on "How Eating Habits Are Formed," eating habits that were developed at an early age tend to stay with us, unless of course we change them. Also, people eat breakfast mainly because they believe that food is required in the mornings to start their engines and keep them running throughout the morning.

You can easily prove false the belief that breakfast is needed by skipping breakfasts entirely, as I do. Try it for several weeks; it usually takes that long to break a habit. See if it doesn't boost your energy levels. I'm confident that you will then look back on your former "breakfast habit" as something that slowed you down for too long.

"The worst and by far the most unhealthy habit is the heavy breakfast. No solid food should be eaten in the early morning at all if you desire to secure the best health results." - Arnold Ehret, *Mucusless Diet Healing System*.

Based on my experience with the raw vegan diet, and with fasting and the no-breakfast plan, I see a lot of truth in the vitality theory. I haven't found much fault in it. Although there appears to be little or no clinical evidence, or proof, as far as I can determine, that vitality is received from an external source/God, anyone who is familiar with miracles realizes that mysterious things can and do happen, and that life itself is a miracle.

Life does not have to be a miserable struggle. Vitality can make all the difference in the world. As mentioned earlier, on the raw vegan diet, you can enjoy a great deal of vitality that others do not have, which enables you to turn many of your struggles into solutions.

"Healthy food gives us the energy to be healthy and happy. When we eat food with energy, we become people with energy. The difference between people with energy and people without energy is quire dramatic." - *Sergei and Valya Boutenko, Eating Without Heating*.

Spirituality

The soul or spirit of man hungers for spiritual sustenance. As the body must be fed with food, so must the soul be fed with spiritual nourishment. Everyone requires this nourishment in their lives, but when we concentrate on other pursuits and neglect the needs of the soul, we become spiritually impoverished. This causes an imbalance in our natures that can felt. It can lead to, among other things, a dissatisfaction and disillusionment about life. St. Augustine of Hippo said that our minds are restless till they rest in Thee. Restlessness reflects our deepest desire for God. Our hearts are restless and they will not rest until they rest in God.

There seems to be little, if any, difference between the soul and spirit of man. Some assume they are the same. The Bible indicates, in Hebrews 4:12, that they are different, although not by much. "For the word of God is quick and powerful, and sharper than any two-edged sword, piercing even to the dividing asunder of soul and spirit, and of the joints and marrow, and is a discerner of the thoughts and intents of the heart."

Similarly, the body and soul of man are bound together in a way that makes them practically inseparable. This is why the seventeenth century theologian, Father Martin Von Cochem, who having had discussions with people who had been raised from the dead, said in his book, *The Four Last Things: Death, Judgement, Hell, Heaven,* that death is a very painful experience since it is when the soul must depart from the body.

Matthew Henry, in his commentary, said that believers are given a measure of the Holy Spirit somewhat as in a vessel of water. But Christ was given the Spirit without measure, as in a fountain or a bottomless ocean. The pain that Jesus experienced when he died on the cross must have been excruciating, as is evidenced from the Gospels by His loud cry right before He gave up His spirit.

We do much to ensure the needs of the soul are well provided for by taking time out of our busy schedules to read the Word of God. The soul also receives nourishment when we pray to God. It is important to pray often, as the apostle Paul tells us, but it is also important to engage in contemplative prayer, a form of prayer that is perhaps best described in William Meninger's *The Loving Search for God.* Remember, an army cannot march on an empty stomach, and the soul must be adequately nourished for spiritual warfare.

Brother Lawrence, in his book, *The Practice of the Presence of God,* says that when we give attention to the Creator, God comes to us in the secret place of the soul. That is a very profound statement. God, who is infinitely perfect in every Divine attribute, including holiness, grace, truth, power, knowledge and love, deigns to have fellowship with redeemed sinners who worship in spirit and in truth, but who are nevertheless full of imperfections and sins. However, it is in weakness that we find strength in Him.

Raw plant foods are known to enhance spirituality in definite ways. As yoga can release blocked chakras and allow the flow of inner energy in the body, so raw plant foods, which help cleanse the body of its toxins, can cause a resurgence of the spirit when the accumulation of toxins is cleared away. Contrarywise, many of the foods that are commonly consumed cause biological disharmony, including pains and discomforts, which distract us from our sources of spiritual sustenance. They are not the foods that should be eaten for tranquility, inner peace and spirituality.

Raw plant foods not only purify the body by enhancing its capacity to absorb vital nutrients, but they also purify the soul by enhancing its capacity for receiving spiritual nourishment.

St. John of the Cross said, "In the state of innocence all that our first parents saw, spoke of, and ate in the garden of paradise served them for more abundant delight in contemplation, since the sensory part of their souls was truly subjected and ordered to reason. The person whose sense is purged of sensible objects and ordered to reason procures from the first movements the delights of savory contemplation and awareness of God."[11]

A Prayer

Father, you have the power to heal all our maladies and resolve all our troubles, but you have given each of us the ability to learn how to do these things ourselves. You lead us and guide us in ways of learning that direct us to the answers we are looking for. You have decreed what foods should be eaten and have given us a plentiful supply of these foods. You are with us in everything that we do. Therefore, we praise you and thank you for all that you have done for us.

---

[11] St. John of the Cross, The Ascent of Mount Carmel, Book 3, Chapter 26.

The Final Hurdle

This chapter covers how to clear the final hurdle to achieve the God-given diet, the raw vegan diet. Assuming the transition period is almost completed, you should be on the vegan diet. To attain the raw vegan diet, a last hurdle remains, the hurdle of overcoming the addiction to cooked foods.

"Our deepest fear is not that we are inadequate. Our deepest fear is that we are powerful beyond measure. It is our light, not our darkness that most frightens us." - Marianne Williamson.

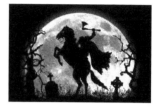

When I was on the vegan diet, I still ate cooked foods. The cooked foods I ate at the time of the final hurdle were canned beans and microwaved sweet potatoes, cabbage, broccoli and carrots. All other foods that I ate were raw fruits and vegetables, leafy greens, nuts and seeds, sea vegetables and Superfoods. The only thing that separated me from being a raw vegan was cooked food.

It was a struggle because my taste buds "knew better" and argued for keeping cooked foods in the diet. It was actually my cravings for cooked foods that stood in the way.

However, before I could get off cooked foods altogether, I had to be fully convinced that they were doing mo harm. I had to understand the dangers that are inherent in eating cooked foods. It was part of my searching for the answers for why my health had reached a standstill and was no longer improving on the vegan diet.

I discovered that the dangers of cooked foods are best elucidated in the books by Norman W. Walker, Arnold Ehret and David Wolfe (see Bibliography). Some of the wisdom contained in these books has been captured in the previous chapters on "The Dangers of Cooked Foods" and "The Dangers of Starchy Foods." If these chapters have not convinced you of the dangers of eating these foods, then you should read the books that are referenced in those chapters. Remember that books are our most trusted source of information about foods and nutrition.

It was the knowledge of the dangers of cooked and starchy foods that enabled me to overcome the strong pulls and ties that these foods have on us. Otherwise, I would still be on the vegan diet, and still hindered by a partially healthy, partially unhealthy diet.

I believe that when you can conceptualize or visualize something, then it has a chance to manifest itself in your life. When I was convinced that cooked foods were harmful to my health, I quit them cold-turkey. It was the application of what I had learned over the power of the cravings I had for these foods. Then, all of a sudden, I was a raw vegan.

However, that did not end the battle that was waging between my taste buds and mind, as I was soon to find out.

My first day on the God-given diet was a red-letter day. I circled it on the calendar. I had at least made the decision to go completely raw.

The very first week of eating only raw plant foods passed quickly and uneventfully, to my great amazement. I was actually doing it; I was making it! I had some minor adjustments to make, to include more living foods in place of the dead foods I had been eating, but everything went well and I was learning more along the way. I circled each day on the calendar as time went by.

I remember it was very exciting. I guess I have always loved new challenges, and this was no exception. Soon, it was two whole weeks of eating only living plant foods. I couldn't believe that I was actually doing it! My self-confidence went up about fifty points.

In the third week of being totally raw, however, intense cravings for cooked foods surfaced and started to really bother me. My mouth would water just thinking about them. I began to second guess this whole raw food thing. After all, why should I give up foods that I really enjoy?? I would take a can of beans and just look at it. I would add more sweet potatoes to my shopping basket just to ensure I had enough at home, in case I started eating them again. It was a struggle that lasted all of the third week and persisted into the fourth week on the God-given diet.

To keep my mind from wondering, I put all cooked food items out of sight and kept the aforementioned books ready at hand, reading them over and over, and continuing to underline sentences that accentuated the dangers of cooked foods.

"When you're going through hell, keep going." - Winston Churchill.

The next thing I knew, a whole month had gone by on the raw vegan diet. The cravings for cooked foods passed along with it.

I discovered it actually was mind over matter, knowledge over desire. And that is how I overcame my cooked food addiction and cleared the hurdle.

I have not returned to cooked foods since and have no intention of doing so. When you are on the whole plant food God-given diet for any length of time, you no longer think about cooked foods. It turns out that nothing you lost was really worth keeping anyway.
How to Quit Cooked Foods

In addition to my own testimony given above, some objective advice and encouragement is warranted.

In order to quit cooked foods, to overcome their addictive power in your life, you must step out of your comfort zone one more time. It requires about the same amount of effort it took to quit meat and dairy products and all sugary foods.

First, there must be a resolve to quit cooked foods based on your self-education and knowledge about foods and nutrition. Then, you must summon the willpower to make it happen.

As mentioned in the chapter on "How Eating Habits are Formed," the so-called cravings of appetite are nothing more than ingrained habits. A habit once acquired and persistently practiced soon becomes a craving. There were no cravings until we acquired and persistently practiced a habit. Cravings stay with us even if they are doing us harm.

Anyone with a little persistence and willpower can change their eating habits, or for that matter any other habit in life. True change always begins in the mind. New eating habits are formed when we accustom the mind to new tastes and food selections based on reason and knowledge rather than emotional pulls and pressures.

"Uncooked foods will supply not only all the necessary vitamins and minerals, but also all the enzymes and easily digestible natural starches and proteins needed for healthy functioning of the body." - Paavo O. Airola, N.D., *There is a Cure for Arthritis.*

Food cravings, habits and addictions that are created or formed when the same foods are habitually eaten, are broken when the foods are continually not eaten. Begin the process by reducing the number of cooked foods in your diet and the frequency of eating them. When you reach a minimum of cooked foods in your diet, strengthen your resolve by reading as much as you can about the dangers of cooked foods and understanding why they are harmful to you.

Effort is required to accomplish anything worthwhile. The dictionary is the only place where success comes before work. Surely, nothing worthwhile in life is ever accomplished without effort, and the things that require the most effort are often the most rewarding and worthwhile of all.

The only way you will ever realize what it takes to quit cooked foods is by actually quitting them. No one can do it for you, it has to be done by you.

As mentioned previously, there is no magic pill or silver bullet for getting well. If you want anything to happen in life, you have to make it happen. That includes quitting cooked foods.

If the raw vegan diet were easy to attain and had zero hurdles to overcome, then more people would be experiencing its remarkable health benefits, and a lot loco of the population would be rushing blindly towards premature graves.

The easy way is always the most traveled, and the difficult way is always the least travelled.

"Enter by the narrow gate; for wide is the gate and broad is the way that leads to destruction, and there are many who go in by it. Because narrow is the gate and difficult is the way which leads to life, and there are few who find it." - Jesus in the Bible, Matt. 7:13-14.

Afterwards

You have now successfully transitioned to the raw vegan diet. Congratulations! You have achieved what few people will ever accomplish. Your determination, discipline and willpower are to be commended. The efforts that you have made will now pay off.

Once the basics of the whole plant food diet are understood (and they are understood when they are put into practice), you have at your disposal the most potent healing and transformational tool ever available. And that is when the adventure really begins.

On a whole plant food diet, self-cleansing is in full gear. The self-cleansing process begins internally and is then reflected externally. This goes against conventional wisdom which says that to be clean all you must do is thoroughly wash with soap and water, but that only contributes to external cleansing. Internal cleansing is necessary to remove the toxins and pasty crud that have accumulated in the organs and tissues of the body from years of eating cooked and starchy foods and other foods and food products that are harmful to health. Normal signs of detoxification, previously discussed, are likely to be experienced, especially as more raw fruits and vegetables are eaten.

The skin, and particularly the skin of the face, reflects our internal health condition. A bad skin complexion (e.g., pimples or blotches on the face) indicates internal poisoning. A clear complexion reveals internal health. It doesn't take long on the raw vegan diet for the skin of the face to clear up, and then become smoother.

It has been reported by some raw food eaters that the face has actually takes on a perceptible glow or shine. This was revealed to me, for example, during a discussion I had with a raw food eater years ago who said he knew a man whose face actually glowed with health. I can't claim glowing skin, but I perceive that it is a possibility. After all, living plant foods provide us with their electric and magnetic properties intact, unaltered by heat. Also, isn't light a manifestation of electromagnetic energy?

Many Medieval and earlier Christian paintings, stained-glass windows and mosaics depict Jesus and the saints with halos over their heads. Could these depictions be based on fact? Arnold Ehret in his book, *The Cause and Cure of Human Illness*, states that many saints of old were self-radiant due to their ascetic diet of raw plant foods and their practice of fasting.

The thought of discovering the "Fountain of Youth" has intrigued many people for centuries, and there have been explorers, such as Ponce de Leon, who have tried to find it. I believe the fountain of youth exists, but not hidden in some distant, exotic land. I believe it is within every person, just waiting to be released through a diet of living plant foods.

Some people spend large amounts of money on beauty products and preparations. If the money were spent instead on self-education about foods and nutrition, and on raw, organic fruits, vegetables, leafy greens and other living plant foods, it would allow health and youthful appearance to be attained without the aid of these products.

Want to look young? Eat raw plant foods. Want to look old? Eat cooked foods.

Health improvements reported by raw food eaters the world over have included not only the complete healing of diseases, but changes indicative of rejuvenation, such as wrinkles disappearing, improved vision, hair growing back and hair color returning to that of former years, among other things. These signs, while seemingly miraculous, are logical consequences of eating living plant foods once you understand the healing powers of these foods. Such improvements are due to the life force in raw plant foods, life force made available to anyone on the raw began diet.

On the raw vegan diet, the body is cleansed not only of poisonous substances that have accumulated over the years and have been deposited deeply in body tissues, but also those that get into the body from the environment, or from foods and drinks, such as chlorine and heavy metals from municipal drinking water, pesticides in non-organic produce, and tobacco and alcohol use.

"Any substance, when taken into the body, is either a food or a poison." - Dr. Herbert M. Shelton, *Superior Nutrition*.

Modern nutritional experts believe that fruits and leafy green vegetables are the greatest cleansers of the body. Both food groups cause toxins to be released from the tissues. The more fruits and leafy greens we eat on a regular basis, the more our internals are scrubbed clean and the more our outward improvements are manifested. Since the self-cleansing process will be on-going from now on, so will visible health improvements.

The effectiveness of the self-cleansing process is also evident by the composition, odor and frequency of stools. Bowel movements become smoother, less smelly and more frequent, which are all signs of internal cleansing becoming a more normal process, and indicating a less clogged up condition due to better digestion and the ongoing removal of poisons from the body. On the raw vegan diet, you may find that the number of bowel movements per day is at least as many as the number of meals eaten per day. Constipation is unknown on the raw vegan diet.

That secret of vitality was explained in the chapter on "Vitality." An abundance of vitality is available to anyone who adopts the raw vegan diet.

The nutritional experts agree that the raw vegan diet, together with fasting, dissolves accumulated toxins better than any other health regimen. When toxins are removed from the body, you feel great.

If you wake up in the mornings feeling groggy, sluggish and in a sour mood, it is probably because of accumulated poisons and waste material that still reside in you, not only in your colon but in the very tissues of your body. These poisons can be adequately purged by eating living plant foods, watching our intake of harmful foods and drinks, performing enemas or colonics and fasting.

The Benefits

Based on my experience and the experiences of others, I believe that the raw vegan diet provides more benefits than have been accounted for or recognized, and that the benefits are boundless, as Nature is boundless.

When I was a vegetarian, and also when I was a vegan, I had health issues that simply could not be shaken. They remained with me until I became a raw vegan. I was plagued with chronic fatigue. I felt worn-out all the time despite getting sufficient sleep. I took organic iron supplements, sublingual vitamin B12 spray, flaxseeds, chia seeds and kelp to counter this condition, but they did not solve the problem.

After being on the raw vegan diet for only a short time, my fatigue vanished into thin air. I now have a surplus of energy. I never have to lie down during the day or take a nap anymore.

"Most persons are tired because their body lacks enzymes. The food they eat cannot be utilized constructively but is turned instead into toxins, poisons which lead to sickness. Enzymes, apparently, are the key to longevity; they seem to neutralize the basic causes of aging and enable the body to retain its youthful qualities." - Dr. Ann Wigmore, *Be Your Own Doctor*.

I attribute the fatigue that I had prior to the raw vegan diet to the lack of enzymes in the cooked foods I was eating.   After several years on the diet, however, I decided it might be wise to take, as a precaution, sublingual vitamin B12 because of the fact that a lack of vitamin B12 is considered a possibility when eating raw plant foods exclusively. But I now never take it.

I had scaly skin on the karate edges of my hands every winter, from November through March. On the raw vegan diet, this condition disappeared.

I'm more physically fit and active now than I've been in years. I lost 14 pounds going from the vegan diet to the raw vegan diet. That's 14 pounds I no longer have to carry around. Also, my vision has improved. I can read books outdoors without corrective lenses. The last time I could do that was in my 40s.

I've had a number of physical ailments including hemorrhoids, sciatica, spinal stenosis and arthritis. But since being on the diet, I have had no further health issues and, of course, no diseases. I cured my hemorrhoids by a simple plant food remedy that is not well known. It is described in the book on hemorrhoids in the Bibliography. I cured my sciatica and spinal stenosis through correction of muscle imbalances as explained in the book on sciatica and spinal stenosis in the Bibliography. I tried so many things to cure my arthritis that I know that the diet, distilled water and intermittent fasting are what have resulted in no more pains.

However, the health improvements I received on the diet pale into insignificance compared to the health improvements experienced by many other raw plant food eaters, including nutritional experts Arnold Ehret, O.L.M. Abramowski, Ann Wigmore, Norman W. Walker, Bernard Jensen, Herbert M. Shelton, Theresa Mitchell, David Wolfe, Professor Spira, Harvey Diamond, Kristina Carrillo-Bucaram, Victoria Boutenko, Tonya Zavasta, and Joe Alexander. Some of these individuals were but a step away from death before they cured themselves of serious chronic diseases through the raw vegan diet. Some also healed themselves of other conditions through the diet, such as bursitis (Tonya Zavasta), and colitis and arthritis (Ann Wigmore). Their testimonies are included in their books listed in the Bibliography. They validate the power of living plant foods to completely heal illnesses and diseases.

I highly recommend the books in the Bibliography just for the testimonies. They will convince you of the importance of eating living plant foods exclusively, and encourage you in the diet.

It may interest you to know that Dr. Norman W. Walker lived to be 99 (according to the Web), but some sources, including David Wolf, say 109. Dr. Herbert M. Shelton lived to be 100. Dr. Bernard Jensen lived to be 93. Dr. Edward Howell lived to 90. Dr. D. C. Jarvis lived to 85. Arnold Ehret died accidentally at 56 when he slipped on a wet, oil-soaked street in California and fell back and hit his head on the payment. Dr. Ann Wigmore died at 85 from smoke inhalation when a fire broke out at her Institute while she was sleeping. Most of the other nutritional experts are still living.

The body is the greatest healing machine. It only requires the right foods to accomplish what it alone knows how to do. When living plant foods are eaten in place of dead, cooked foods, the body receives the amazing ionic and magnetic properties of living foods as well as their potent, unaltered natural minerals, vitamins and enzymes.

The on-going self-cleansing of the body that is achieved by eating living plant foods exclusively is complemented by another process, one also on-going. That process is the cellular reconstruction of the body.

The body is constantly replacing its cells. Old cells are being replaced by new cells. The difference between the raw vegan diet and other diets is that on the raw vegan diet the body is provided with the best raw materials for this reconstruction process.

When we eat cooked foods including refined and processed man-made foods, which are dead foods, the new cells are constructed of inferior quality building materials.

"Dead atoms and dead molecules cannot rejuvenate or regenerate the cells of the body. Such food results in cell starvation and this in turn causes sickness and disease." - Dr. Norman W. Walker, *Water Can Undermine Your Health*.

The time required for cellular reconstruction varies depending on the organs and tissues of the body. The following information is taken from the Web.

AVERAGE BODY CELL REPLACEMENT TIME

- White blood cells   2-5 days

- Stomach cells   2-9 days

- Lung alveoli   8 days

- Trachea cells   1-2 months

- Red blood cells   5 months

- Skeleton cells   10% p.a.

This indicates that after only a short time, the body has replaced many of its cells, and if we are on the raw vegan diet the new cells have been made from the best raw materials of life, those found in living plant foods. The longer we eat raw foods exclusively, the more we are being reconstructed from the materials provided by living plant foods.

It requires years for the body to replace all of its cells (which number some ten trillion), but, in time, they all get replaced -- at least the vast majority of them do as far as we know. It is uncertain whether all the neurons of the brain get replaced.

Some scientists believe that at any one time in a person's life, the cells and tissues of the body are no more than 7 years old. If true, it sets a short-term goal for all of us on the raw vegan diet, which is to remain on the diet for at least 7 years to be totally reconstructed from the best raw materials of Nature.

The new you is in the making, and you are able to sense it, and that alone makes each day a new experience. You are being transformed inside out, and if you pause for a moment during your busy day to think about it, it just may put a smile on your face.

As discussed previously, the raw vegan diet provides all the vitamins, proteins, and other nutrients required to attain and sustain a healthy life. However, some raw foodists have reported a deficiency of vitamin B-12. There are few plant foods that contain vitamin B-12. To be on the safe side, you can take a vitamin B-12 supplement in the form of an organic sublingual spray, which is available at whole food stores. As with all of the B vitamins, vitamin B-12 is water soluble and flushes out of the system if more is taken than the body can use. You can also take an organic iron supplement to help avoid fatigue.

If you take supplements, you should ensure that they are in organic, not inorganic, form. As explained previously, the cells of the body utilize minerals that are in organic form, which is one of the reasons that plant foods are so important to us. Plants convert the inorganic minerals found in the soil and water into organic form that is readily assimilated by the body.

A noticeable improvement occurred after time on the diet. My senses of smell and taste became keener, which helped me to refine and improve my diet, such as by eating more nutritious raw plant foods and avoiding ones not so nutritious.

The only "shock" I experienced on the raw vegan diet occurred several months into the diet. I noticed many large wrinkles on my skin, especially on the face and the back of the neck. My immediate reaction was, what is going on? So once again, I went to books for the answers. I discovered that this occurrence is normal on the raw vegan diet, and that it soon passes. It is reflective of the detoxification process and indicates the success of it. Teresa Mitchell explains this in her book, *My Road to Health*. She states that it is a normal sign of the healing process that is going on. The wrinkles go away and skin elasticity returns when the blood and tissues are rebuilt using the optimum building blocks of living natural foods. And that is exactly what happened to me.

As for habits such as alcohol and tobacco, the diet will eventually cause the body to reject what is bad for it. If you have difficulty quitting such habits, then let the diet handle it for you.

SAY GOODBYE TO THESE THINGS

- Microwave Oven

- Stove

- Baking Accessories

- Pots and Pans

- Cooking Utensils

- Can Openers

- Popcorn Maker

- Toaster

- Rice Cooker

The same week I quit cooked foods and became a raw vegan, I gave away my microwave oven. By giving it away, I burned a bridge to my past that I never want to cross again. When I was convinced of the harmful effects that cooked foods have on the body, I wanted to be not only free of cooked foods, but of all the devices or gadgets I possessed which were used in connection with cooked foods.

Getting rid of the microwave oven and the other cooking tools and utensils was my declaration of independence on the raw vegan diet. It cemented my resolve to stick with the diet.

The stove, because of its bulk and weight, was more difficult to give away, so I kept it. It now has a large cutting board spanning the upper burners. I sometimes use the oven in winter to help heat up the kitchen. Otherwise, it goes unused.

In addition, canned, bottled or jarred food products in the kitchen cabinets can now be given away or donated to the local food banks, many of which are supported by local churches that have drop off centers you can use.

The new-found space in the kitchen can then be put to better use for storage of raw food items, such as containers of nuts and seeds, sun-dried fruits and Superfoods.

Specific Benefits of the Raw Vegan Diet

Some of the benefits of the raw vegan diet have already been described. Below is a more complete list. These benefits have been experienced by raw food eaters in every generation the world over, including myself and the authors of the books that are listed in the Bibliography. The benefits are all extraordinary in their own way. Some are experienced after only a short time on the diet.

- Heals diseases

- Prevents diseases from taking root in the body

- Rejuvenates and beautifies

- Increases energy

- Promotes health and longevity

- Reduces weight

- Improves mental clarity

- Adds excitement to life

- Improves decision making

- Improves sleeps

- Makes you feel good about being alive

Let's examine two that have not yet been discussed.

Let's take the last benefit first. How many people do you know, or see every day, who have a frown on their face? How many times can that be said of you? Our general health affects the way that we feel, which often results in a display of outward signs. When we are healthy, we feel good about being alive and tend to show it. When we're unhealthy, we tend to show that too.

As discussed in the chapter on "Spirituality," raw plant foods enhance the spirit in definite ways, charging or supercharging it. After about a year on the diet you will find yourself paying more attention to the spiritual aspects of life, and praying more often and earnestly than you did before because you are now more thankful for being alive.

The healing of diseases is the most significant benefit that can be expected on the raw vegan diet. As explained previously, healing is achieved by eating living raw plant foods exclusively, adopting proper eating habits, and performing fasting. It is the natural consequence of the on-going cellular reconstruction process utilizing the best building materials found in Nature, and the bodily detoxification process that follows.

"All illnesses, including the inherited diseases, stem from biologically wrong, unnatural food, and from every gram of excess food intake. The exceptions are rare, e.g., lack of hygiene." - Arnold Ehret, *The Mucusless Diet Healing System*.

How long does it take for healing to occur on the raw vegan diet? According to the nutritional experts, it depends on how long one has been eating harmful foods. Many people have neglected their health for years before becoming a raw vegan.

The healing process can be speeded up depending on what is done to assist it. For example, if you periodically fast and perform colonics and/or enemas, then quicker results can be expected. If you do not do these things, then delayed results can be expected. But the important thing is, the healing process begins in earnest when you are committed to the raw vegan diet.

David Wolfe in his book, *The Sunfood Diet Success System,* states that it typically takes one month on the diet to reverse one year on a cooked/toxic food diet, to dissolve and eliminate the improper materials that have accumulated in the body. But this schedule, apparently, does not consider the accelerators of periodic fasting and colonics and/or enemas.

The excitement builds as progress becomes more noticeable on the diet. For example, in a very short time on the raw vegan diet you will begin to lose weight. Also, your complexion will clear up. Other encouraging rejuvenation signs will appear as well.

Expect to have a surplus of energy that enables you to do more things. Expect to be able to work and play without tiring.

You will begin to function at an enhanced awareness level. Your senses of sight, sound, smell and taste will become more acute, or heightened.

You will have a clarity of mind that will enable you to make right decisions.

You will sense that more health improvements are on the way. You realize that the days ahead are going to be better than the days behind. Isn't that how you want to start every day of your life?

As the health improvements become more apparent, you will be able to gauge your progress. But, however long it takes, do not give up.

The more you can hone, or attune, the diet to the preferences of the body, the healthier you will become, and the sharper your mind will become. In particular, you learn to avoid foods that are difficult to digest.

"As your body becomes smarter and more accustomed to the changes you are introducing, it will direct you toward consuming less food, and that food will be of the very best quality. No matter how incredible it might sound to a beginner, the day will come when you will no longer care for recipes. At first you cannot stand the lightness that consumption of raw foods produces, but after several years on this lifestyle it is fullness that becomes insufferable." - Tonya Zavasta, *Beautiful on Raw Uncooked Creations*.

I am more convinced now than ever before that the most beneficial plant foods, those that contribute most to the healing process and to optimum health, are the foods that are the most "alive," that is, foods that have been the most recently harvested.

Many, if not all, of the raw plant foods that are sold in local food stores have been harvested more than a week ago (unless grown locally). They have been shipped-in from faraway places in an un-ripened condition, which typically means that they have been in cold storage for weeks. They have been sprayed with wax to retard spoilage. They have been labeled. Most appear to be flawless copies of one other, uniform in size, shape and color.

Locally grown and/or Community Supported Agriculture (CSA) farm produce is organically grown produce. The farms are typically family owned and operated, or non-profit organizations. The produce is typically no more than a few days old from being harvested at peak ripeness. It hasn't been labelled or sprayed with wax. CSA fruits and vegetables are not necessarily uniform in appearance, but they typically have flaws. Their life-giving properties have been least altered or affected by the growers and the suppliers.

I benefit from a CSA and recommend everyone do the same. If you happen to live in a country other than the US, there should be a local food producer and supplier in your area where fresh produce is available.

In my opinion, the further away we get from the heavy use of herbicides and pesticides in the many large-scale factory farms, the prematurely harvested foods that are shipped-in from long distances, such as from China, South America and Africa, and the various cosmetic measures that have been applied to them to make them more appealing to the sight, the better off we will be as consumers of fruits, vegetables and other raw foods, and the quicker we will experience the benefits of the raw vegan diet.

"I believe that family farms ought to be considered our greatest natural resource, and that the fundamental healthfulness of our food and the long-term health of our economy are closely tied to their well-being." - Howard F. Lyman, *Mad Cowboy.*

The nutritional advantages of eating locally grown produce over other produce have been covered in the chapter on "The Foods We Should Eat and Why."

Most of us lack the yard space for planting a garden, and only few of us will ever be able to afford a farm. The closest most of us will ever get to locally grown produce is by joining a CSA.

We have spent too much time and effort learning about the foods of the animal kingdom and how to prepare them. It is time we learned about the foods of the plant kingdom and the many tasty and nutritious meals that can be made from them. Each kind of living plant food has its own unique blend of nutrients and life-giving properties. We can benefit from eating many types of raw plant foods. I believe that the vast variety of plant foods in the world have been given to us for a purpose, and that we can discover that purpose by becoming familiar with these foods.

An aspect of a whole plant food diet that strikes me as being most interesting is that it doesn't leave you guessing about whether your health is going to improve. Your health does not stall or level-off and then decline on the diet, as it does on other diets. It continues to improve. Each day on the diet is an ongoing progression, a new adventure, sometimes trying until the key points discussed in this book are mastered, but never a losing proposition. Each day that you are on the diet you are a winner.

A new story is being written. It is a story that continues to be written as long as you remain on the living food, raw vegan diet. It is a story about you -- the new you. Maybe it is the best story ever.

A Simpler Life

"Health is Nature's reward for getting into harmony with her laws."
- Alfred Armand Montapert.

A simpler life is what we all yearn for, a life that has less worries, less cares and less stresses. But how can it be attained? How can we live a life that is less discordant with Nature, our true mother, that recognizes life as the miracle it is, yet acknowledging how fragile and transitory it is? What is the secret?

Remember, "...the simplicity that is in Christ..." - 2 Cor. 11:3.

In my opinion, the raw vegan diet is one of the keys to a simpler life. It has proven to be the best diet for restoring health, healing diseases, rejuvenating the body and attaining optimum health. As explained in this book, the conditions required for ill-health cannot exist in a body that has cleansed itself of toxic wastes through the powers of living plant foods. When we are no longer burdened by ill-health conditions, when we are freed from their many demands and constraints on our efforts and time, we begin to smell the roses, notice the finer things in life and live a simpler life. But only a few of us will ever adopt the raw vegan diet. If more of us were to do so, the suffering that is in the world and in most people's lives would be much less than it is today.

The world is daily becoming more and more complex, and complexity is the opposite of simplicity. Its complexity is like a runaway train that has no breaks. It is drifting further and further away from God and a simple, natural life.

With all the problems that confront us, and the many pulls and pressures that are on our lives, we hardly have time to do anything we really want to do. Trampled by cares and worries, and vexed by the many things that wreck our peace and quiet, it is a wonder that any of us can keep our heads above the waves.

Many people work long hours in order to earn a living. I used to be one of them. The time remaining each day is typically reserved for meals and whatever relaxation or amusement can be squeezed in. In the attempt to balance the equation, many of us resort to health-destroying habits, such as consuming refined and processed foods and drinks, and overeating. A means of escaping the confusion and frustration of everyday life is frequently sought through food and drink preferences. Anything is tried that would help to blot out the nagging reality of an unhappy existence.

Meanwhile, our souls cry out for simplicity, for inner peace, for less pressures and stresses, for time to do more important things and experience life as perhaps it should be experienced, as a meaningful joy. Consider what the Bible says about the early Christians.

"So continuing daily with one accord in the temple, and breaking bread from house to house, they ate their food with gladness and simplicity of heart, praising God and having favor with all the people." - Acts 2:46-47.

Does that describe most of us?

As citizens of the most influential economic and military power in the world, we ought to be contented people. But discontent is everywhere. To rest in the simple pleasures and joys that life has to offer is something that very few of us will ever experience, even those who have wealth beyond measure.

Outside influences often cause the struggles that we have. A peaceful, quiet life in the country is not attainable for everybody, but such a life is known to be much more conducive to health and well-being than living in the city with its many noises, people and distractions. It is difficult today to escape from unwanted sounds.

Eckhart Tolle tells us in his book, *The Power of Now*, that in every life situation there are three choices or options that are available to us. We can remove ourselves from the situation, we can change the situation, or we can accept the situation. The raw vegan diet enables us to change much of the situation. To begin living a simpler life, we need to eat foods that are proven to be healthy for us and avoid the foods that are harmful to us.

A great conformity has dropped over this country. It is no doubt due, at least in part, to education by popular media and the regimentation of social life. By putting material things in the forefront of our lives, many of us have neglected the more important matters of life, such as family, inner peace, and health and well-being. As far as foods and drinks are concerned, many people in this country know more about the latest "energy drink" than they do about raw plant foods, and care little for deviating from what they have grown accustomed to eat and drink.

Bad diet is fast becoming the number one cause of death in this country and throughout the world. When we realize how commonly consumed foods harm us and start eating healthier foods, we avoid many of the sicknesses and diseases that are attributed to bad diet, such as heart disease, kidney disease, diabetes and cancer of the organs, to name just a few.

Many people do not realize how their health influences their feelings about life. As explained in the chapter on "Afterwards," if you wake up feeling groggy, sluggish and in a sour mood, you may not know why but the cause very likely lies within. It is probably due to the accumulated toxins and waste matter that reside within you, not only in the colon but in the very tissues of your body, toxins that have not yet been purged by the body's self-cleansing process. The biological disharmony that this creates is most evident first thing in the morning.

The disharmony felt in the mornings can be caused by what we ate the day before or the night before, or by how we ate it. A way of life discordant with the laws of Nature destroys the harmony of the organism. Likewise, a way of life in harmony with her laws preserves the harmony of the organism.

Peace of mind and worry-free existence are possible. All it takes is the willingness to alter certain things about our lives and the discipline to carry it out. Upon our death, let not our life be summed up as follows (gender not important), "May he rest in peace, he found little of it while he was alive."

I am not alone when I say that I do not want to spend the rest of my days in disharmony with Nature and her laws, nor do I intend to let it happen. The consequences of being in disharmony with nature, such as being in the throes of pain or drugged by medication and robbed of health, does not have to be anyone's fate. We now have at our disposal the practical know-how to change these things.

As discussed previously, a fundamental law of nature is the law of cause and effect. When we eat foods that are harmful to the body, or are improperly combined, or consume too much food too often, we invite the inevitable consequences of ill-health. To avoid these consequences, we must do the things that promote and sustain health. It is up to us to live more in harmony with nature. Perhaps the initial step to optimum health is accepting full responsibility for our health. It is a step that many people will never take, except maybe when it is too late for it to make any difference. The choice is ours.

"It is not enough that we do our best; sometimes we must do what is required." - Winston Churchill.

The foods that are best for health are those that have their vital nutrients and enzymes intact (the body requires nutrients, and enzymes to break down the nutrients, for foods to be properly assimilated in the body). These are the foods as-found in nature, replete with their life-giving properties. These are the foods of the raw vegan diet.

A simpler life is obtained by doing the things that are described in this book, including adopting the raw vegan diet, learning to properly combine foods, learning proper eating habits, assisting the internal cleansing process by performing colonics, enemas and/or fasting, and getting the proper amount of exercise and rest.

How to Be Your Own Doctor

The best way to reach health goals is to take charge of your own health and learn how to be your own doctor. Nobody is born with knowledge; it must be gained. When the knowledge required to promote and sustain health is gained and put into practice, practically any health issue that assails us can be effectively dealt with without the doctors' advice. It equips us to become, in many ways, our own doctors. This reality has far reaching consequences for our health and well-being, providing numerous health benefits, and preventing numerous health disorders.

The more we learn about foods and nutrition, how to detoxify the body, how to properly combine foods, etc., the more we become our own doctors. It is then that we can resolve our own health issues, and often in ways that completely surprise us. One day they're there, and a few days later they're gone. It is all due to the amazing powers of living plant foods to cleanse the body of its impurities and restore us to health.

The process proceeds something like this. Health improvements begin with the clear realization that a healthy diet must be embraced, which is gained by a knowledge of foods and nutrition. Then comes the somewhat harder part, putting into practice what has been learned. But it gets easier as we experience health improvements as the body rids itself of accumulated toxins, and as we fine-tune the diet based on feedback from the body.

The body is much wiser than we may think it is. It affects the mind so significantly that it may be said to control the mind. Eating a whole plant food diet results in genuine health, which profoundly affects the mind by increasing mental stamina and clarity.

The health corner is turned when we give up foods that are harmful to the body and eat foods that promote health. There is something about eating raw plant foods that strikes a chord of recognition deep within us, as though we intuitively know that these foods are best for us.

Health improvements can occur overnight, but they typically take time. Nature is not on the 9:15 PM express to the suburbs. She does not rush, but takes her time as necessary to complete her work. The damage done to the system by years of unintentional wrong eating requires correction by the body's self-cleansing process before improvements are noticeable.

"Nature takes her time to heal and cure, but the results are lasting. When people appreciate this, and try it, they learn that Nature wants man to live a life of simplicity. It is man who makes life complicated." - Dr. Norman W. Walker.

Since health conditions are quickly resolved on a whole plant food diet, the time and money saved on doctors and prescriptions can be used for other things. Energy levels increase and health cares no longer burden us.

Being your own doctor has advantages besides saving money on hospital stays and doctor bills. The sense of accomplishment and the boost in self-esteem that follows being able to heal yourself of a health issue are priceless rewards. Is there a doctor in the house? Yes, and it's you!

What is better for the budget than raw fruits and vegetables? When we purchase refined and processed foods, we are paying a premium for what was done to them. In comparison, natural foods are much less expensive. Local food stores typically sell onions for under a dollar a pound, and a large cluster of garlic cloves for about half a dollar. Onions and garlic are marvelous foods, and do not have to be purchased organic. A large bunch of carrots, two heads of cabbage, a head of cauliflower, several onions, a cluster of celery, some lemons and a bunch of bananas typically costs less than 10 USD, and may last for more than a week.

Stay with the diet and you will reap the benefits of it. Give up during times of disappointment or frustration, and all will be lost. Remember that if the attainment of genuine health required no knowledge or effort or discernment whatsoever on the part of an individual, then everyone would be remarkably healthy.

Being our own doctor in essence means learning all you can about foods and nutrition from informed sources, such as the books that are referenced in the Bibliography, putting into practice what you learn from these sources, and heeding the signals the body gives about what should and should not be eaten.

"Life's greatest achievement is the continual remaking of yourself so that at last you know how to live." - Winfred Rhodes.

Natural cures have one thing in common, they aim at correcting the underlying causes of health disorders instead of suppressing the symptoms.

Nature

A great contributor to the quality of a healthier, simpler and more enjoyable life is the time spent outdoors in nature.

Almost all of our lives (think of it!) are spent indoors. We "live" in offices and homes, typically under 9- or 10-foot ceilings, in controlled environments of artificial light, heat, humidity and air conditioning, with little fresh air provided. This type of living is more confinement than liberty. It creates subtle but harmful effects on mind and body, such as prevailing undercurrents of vexation, or a feeling that something isn't quite right, and so tension builds.

The time that most people spend outdoors is limited to walking to and from their cars or some form of public transportation.

It is healthy to be outdoors in nature, but not if all we do is walk to and from our cars or the bus or train stop. In order to experience the health benefits that nature has to offer, we need to spend more time out in nature than most of us do. Even a walk in the rain, a bike ride in the park or a climb up a hill helps us to experience, and benefit from, nature.

A Christian Diet

People who make it a habit to spend time outdoors enjoy the refreshing liberty it provides. Nature is not confined or restricted in breadth, width, height or depth as homes and offices are. Birds fly wherever they want. The wind comes and goes wherever it wishes. Sunlight is not artificial, but pure, full spectrum luminosity with all the wavelengths man was intended to receive.

Sunshine has always been a great healer and purifier. It is a natural remedy for many skin conditions. It relaxes the nerves and reduces stress. It acts as a tonic on the immune system.

When we get plenty of sunshine, we enjoy life more, not only because of the vitamin D it provides, but for the healthy complexion and positive attitude that it gives us. A lack of sunshine has the opposite effect. A lack of sunshine has been attributed to the depression experienced by people who live in colder climates, who stay indoors during the winter months.

As cloudy days make us feel glum, sunny days make us feel like getting out of doors because of the life force that is in sunshine.

If you are partial to sweet fruits, then you should get more sunshine because, according to nutritionists, fruit acts as a natural insulin, which lowers blood sugar levels.

When was the last time you viewed the stars? The stars and the constellations in the heavens are difficult to see in our crowded cities and neighborhoods, but by not looking up we miss out on a part of the created world that was provided for our edification.

As we spend more time outdoors, we become more in tune with nature. We discover new things about ourselves, things that would not have come to light in any other way. Nature is a living organism, as the term Mother Nature implies. We share many things in common with her, who reveals to us the simple fact that development and growth are normal, natural processes, and that everything unfolds to fulfill its purpose in life.

Spending time outdoors has a calming effect on the mind. Just viewing the horizon can be very relaxing and gratifying, and inspiring.

"When in despair, one look at a glorious sunset will provide the will to go on." - Franklin Delano Roosevelt.

When we are in harmony with nature, things are better for us, and that is when we can best fulfill our purpose in life. When our conditions are suitable for health, growth and development, when the right "soil" and other factors are present for health and well-being, our purpose becomes clarified. Perhaps not really before then, not when there is so much separation between us and nature.

Unlike the rest of nature, we have been given a free will to determine what is best for us. The rest of nature works only on the level of basic drives, instincts, emotions and passions. But our free will enables us to transcend these things. Free will defines us, it epitomizes us. However, when the gift is not properly used, it can cause us much harm. The more we adhere to our basic drives, instincts, emotions and passions, the more difficult life is for us. But the more we transcend these things by properly using our free will, the more we are the glory of creation.

"A man who has a great attachment to rich foods, in spite of the fact that they may be very unhealthy for him, demeans himself and lowers himself from the status of a noble, intellectual creature formed in the image of God to an animal lusting for material pleasure." - St. John of the Cross.

All phenomena we observe in nature, including the weather, gravity, electricity, chemical reactions and life and death itself, are to some extent mysterious, because Nature does not easily reveal her secrets. Her secrets must be acquired through efforts, by using our minds and abilities to figure out how these things occur so we can use them for our benefit.

But regardless of what our understanding of these things may be, the wonder of nature remains, and, in my opinion, will always remain because man's understanding of his natural world is always limited. Even today, not a single natural phenomenon is fully understood by humankind.

Take, for example, electricity. Nikola Tesla (1856-1943), inventor of the alternating current (AC) motor, believed that electricity came from the air, and that the atmosphere, being electrically charged by the sun (as evidenced by lightning and the auroras), provides the free electrons. Modern engineers, however, believe that electricity is produced, or generated, by power plants through the action of steam on turbine wheels which spin rotors that are within stators. Tesla knew that you cannot create energy out of nothing, but modern engineers seem to have lost sight of that fact.

Another example is the ever-changing weather. It seems to have a mind of its own. Even with advanced computers supposedly capable of very exacting weather forecasts, predicting the weather is no more of a science today than is fishing, and forecasters are known to be notoriously unreliable.

"In all the things that so great and wise a God has created, there must be many secrets." - St. Teresa of Avila.

Self-forgiveness

We need to forgive ourselves, because we are all imperfect in thought, word and deed. We are taught to forgive others, but rarely, if ever, to forgive ourselves, which is equally, if not more, important. When was the last time you forgave yourself?

If you have experienced a serious loss, setback or unexpected and costly turn of events (and who hasn't), it makes no sense to continue to criticize yourself for it, or be angry with yourself for your ignorance or failure in allowing it to happen. It only makes matters worse. Bad things happen to everyone. To err is human. Our physical and mental well-being during times of loss often depend on how we view and treat ourselves.

An authentic acceptance of the facts, including the reasons for their being, is, at times, not only the best thing to do but the only thing to do.

We need to train ourselves to be more forgiving of ourselves, to be more detached instead of on top of ourselves all the time. Seeing ourselves more from an infinite perspective rather than a finite one is a result of seeing ourselves more objectively. It is then that we begin to acknowledge that everything is a lesson, a way of strengthening us.

Miracles

Miracles occur around us every day that are often overlooked and rarely appreciated. Thoughts control our reality. When we think about miracles, positive thoughts replace negative and troubling thoughts, and the more we think about miracles, the more the many stresses and worries of life diminish in intensity.

There are plenty of miracles to think about. That cut on the finger, how miraculously it heals itself. Or the way the body knows only by taste or smell what digestive juices to use for foods. Would these things be easy to program a computer to do?

Or take the parable of the mustard seed. The tiny seed contains the potential not only for growing into a large plant but for producing many more plants. A seed is infinity in living form.

Consider how clouds can store the essence of hundreds of gallons of water aloft, yet do not fall crashing to the earth. They are amazing wonders of creation. The same goes for the many other marvelous phenomena that make up the natural beauty of the created world.

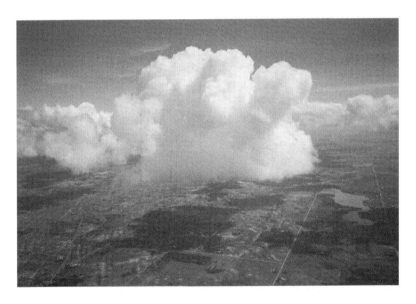

"He binds up the water in His thick clouds, yet the clouds are not broken under it." - Job 26:8.

A Christian Diet

Our very existence is a miracle. Our introduction into this world is shrouded in mystery, as is our introduction into the spiritual world. Who can sufficiently understand these things? Charles Spurgeon once said that no one can explain how the Spirit of God breathes into the soul the breath of spiritual life.

Many people believe that Nature and God are synonymous, that God is in the rocks, the trees and in all living things. It is a belief that is fostered by pantheism or deism. The Bible reveals that God resides in heaven ("Our Father, who is in heaven...").

St. John of the Cross, who is considered by many to be one of the most insightful of the saints, stated, "God sustains every soul and dwells in it substantially, even though it may be that of the greatest sinner in the world. This union between God and creatures always exists. By it, He conserves their being so that if the union should end they would immediately be annihilated and cease to exist." - St. John of the Cross, Book 2, Chapter 5, *The Ascent of Mount Carmel.*

While God and creation are distinct from one another, all of creation is sustained by God. I think of God's sustaining power in the breath of life He gives to all creatures, which we have until we die, and in His power to keep the atoms of all molecules from imploding into themselves by the electrical attraction the electrons have for the oppositely charged protons in the nucleus. Many physicists have been searching intently for this mysterious power, or force, for years, but to no avail.

The apostle Paul, speaking in the Areopagus in Athens, said, "And He has made from one blood every nation of men to dwell on all the face of the earth, and has determined their preappointed times and the boundaries of their dwellings, so that they should seek the Lord, in the hope that they might grope for Him and find Him, though He is not far from each one of us; for in Him we live and move and have our being..." - Acts 17:26-29.

The distinction between God and Nature is also made in the book, *The Essene Gospel of Peace*, which was described in a previous chapter.

On the God-given diet, we learn how the foods of nature bestow health and happiness on poor souls. We begin to view many things in a brighter perspective. As a result, life becomes more enjoyable and we become more appreciative of the little things life has to offer, many of which are normally overlooked.

Fresh fruits and vegetables become more treasured, as does pure water, fresh air and sunshine. We become more aware of how the body is wonderfully and marvelously made. As the Psalmist said, "Marvelous are Your works, O Lord, and that my soul knows very well." - Ps. 139:14.

At sunrise or sunset, go to where you can see the sun moving against the horizon. My mother once told me this. Then she showed me a sunset and said, "This is who we are." And I understood what she meant; that we are all part of the created world.

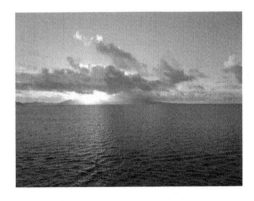

Other Factors

Optimum health is primarily attained by adopting the raw vegan diet and learning proper food combinations and eating habits. It is aided by a number of health-orientated living practices, such as periodic, or intermittent, fasts, drinking distilled water, and using the right kind of salt. The more we are eating living plant foods, using our free will to improve our health rather than destroy it, and turning our thoughts to the wonders of the created world, the healthier we become. But other factors also come into play, and they are discussed in this chapter.

Exercise

Our lives have a physical component. We must not neglect getting the physical exercise we need to maintain health.

We have a cultural propensity for living a sedentary lifestyle. We live in an age of affordable computer-based information and learning tools that enable us to quickly gain access to many subjects, including those that involve entertainment, medical care, shopping, communication, home living, recreation and transportation. Our entire economy, including the government and military, are utterly dependent on computers and will continue to be so. However, computers, whether mainframes, desktops, laptops or smart phones, greatly contribute to a sedentary lifestyle. It is sometimes difficult to leave a computer for any length of time, and cell phones are a constant distraction. The more time we spend sitting down, the more our muscles, tendons and ligaments become adjusted to a sitting posture.

The gluteal (buttocks), leg and abdominal muscles, as well as other muscles of the body become weakened by a sedentary lifestyle. Everyone needs these muscles for certain tasks and activities, but rarely, or maybe never, do the majority of us walk or run fast enough, or do other physical activities, that effectively exercises them. For example, the slower we walk, the less these muscles are used. If we never "rise to the occasion" or get up quickly out of a chair, these muscles may never be effectively used at all, which means that they just atrophy and become ineffective.

Muscle imbalances can wreck your health. For example, they can produce the dreadful pains of sciatica and spinal stenosis, as explained in the book on sciatica and spinal stenosis that is listed in the Bibliography.

Yoga helps to stretch muscles, tendons and ligaments and keep them from atrophying. Yoga is recommended for all ages, but it is particularly recommended for those who are advanced in age. Yoga takes the path of most resistance. A loss of flexibility is a sign of old age, but not for people who practice yoga.

I've been a yoga practitioner for years, first learning the various poses designed to help relieve low back pain, and then progressing to poses that are intended to help sciatica and other physical ailments, and I can testify to the power of yoga to help correct the muscle imbalances caused by a sedentary lifestyle.

Weight training is very helpful for all ages too, as is swimming, running, biking and jogging. They increase bone density and improve the ability to perform normal activities. They keep the blood moving and the muscles toned.

Exercise improves sleep. It helps us to breathe deeper and work out the lungs. It strengthens the cardiovascular system. Exercise is known to improve mood and reduce feelings of depression and anxiety.

Harvey Diamond in his books (two of which are listed in the Bibliography) tells us that exercise is important for the lymph system which has no pump similar to the cardiovascular system's heart to pump the lymph fluid. The lymph system is stimulated by exercise. It is crucial for proper immune system functioning.

Exercise also serves as a healthy stress-reliever, allowing adrenaline that is often secreted into our systems from pent-up emotions such as anger, frustration and bitterness, to be eliminated. Exercise allows us the opportunity to take it out on the weights or the track instead of others.

Rest and Relaxation

Rest and relaxation are crucial for overcoming health problems. As shown throughout this book, when the body is pushed too hard for too long it will not adequately function, and something eventually breaks down. Healing is not possible without adequate rest.

As we take on more and more obligations and objectives, stress can build up to intolerable levels. Handling stress in healthful ways is difficult in our culture since there are so many surrogate stress relievers available.

Nervous disorders resulting from overwork are very common in the Western world. Nervous strain can last for years before a mental or physical breakdown occurs. I know because it happened to me. I was pushing myself relentlessly for over 20 years until I was wrecked by nervous strain and had to take a long break from work to recuperate.

Nervous disorders contribute to illness and disease. It is known that stress causes constriction of the muscle tissues and eliminative organs which results in the retention of metabolic waste, or constipation. Stress also causes a depletion of calcium, magnesium and zinc, minerals that we need for health. As mentioned previously, stress produces acidity in the body, and research has shown that mental stress is one of the highest causes of free radical activity in the body.

Sometimes you can fight too hard. There are times when it pays to rest and take it easy, maybe for a week or even for a day. For leaders of large corporations who have had open heart surgery and who have thought about *walking* out and giving it all up, but have then relented and returned to work, it is only a matter of time before they are *carried* out.

Medication is widely prescribed, and taken, for nervous conditions, but no drug can cure a nervous disorder. You can cope with stress through medication, but you cannot get rid of it that way.

The best way to handle stress is through rest and relaxation. The remedy is so simple that it is generally overlooked, but it's true.

The Bible teaches us that rest and relaxation is vital to well-being. The Sabbath day was given to Israel not for their punishment but for their health and well-being. God knew that we needed rest. He felt so strongly about it that the observance of the Sabbath day was a commandment.

It is said that worry is a dividend paid to disaster before it happens. Worry is wasted energy. Hurry, worry and tension take an enormous toll in this society. They age a person fast. We need to pause more often and take time out for rest and relaxation before we wear ourselves out. But many people feel that taking a "time out" or pausing for breaks or rests is one of the hardest challenges they face. I know, it was true for me not long ago.

"It is not only fun to just do nothing, it is healthful and necessary." - Paul C. Bragg.

The world is very distracting to our senses. It's easy to become overwhelmed by the barrage of its sounds, images and suggestions. One way is to leave the TV and radio off. Another is to read more books about foods and nutrition and not put it off until one has free time, which never comes. Also, leave the cell phone off.

Prayer and Meditation

"The best cure for the body is a quiet mind." - Napoleon Bonaparte.

Prayer and meditation are very beneficial for health and well-being. For Christians, meditation is somewhat the same as prayer, but not so for non-Christians. Both practices have a quieting effect on mind and body. The time spent in prayer or meditation should be at least long enough to produce this quieting effect.

For Christians, prayer has more important benefits, for prayer is the knock that opens the door to heaven.

Prayer may be prompted by feelings of gratitude, or desperation, pain, or the need to plead for deliverance from whatever is bothering us. Prayer requires faith in God, but meditation does not. But both prayer and meditation, especially Transcendental Meditation, relax the mind and body, and enhance clear thinking and well-being.

The health benefits of prayer and meditation include stress reduction, reduced blood pressure, improved sleeps, and relief from anxiety. Both are known to lower hormone levels, limit the exasperating fight-or-flight response, lower free radical activity and increase alpha-wave brain activity. They decrease the biological cost of anger, wrath, frustration, bitterness and hardship that negatively impacts the heart, arteries and immune system.

We have very active minds. Thoughts never leave us alone. We are thinking about something all the time, and typically worrying about something. "Martha, Martha, you are worried and troubled about many things" (Luke 10:41) captures the state of mind that most of us are in all the time. Many of our thoughts are stressful and harmful to us. We need a break from their devilish interference in our peace and tranquility. By giving our problems to the Lord, we trust in their eventual resolution, and this has a cathartic effect on the mind.

If it were not for taking these "time outs" from daily struggles, we would be swamped and continually irked by the many stresses that are imposed on us. Stresses can cause one to dwell inordinately in the past or the future, with the mind replaying the same tapes on what we should have done or said; or what may happen next.

When we focus our attention on the Infinite, a profound peace descends upon us. It leads not only to the momentary relief of worry and stress, but to improved mental health and emotional stability. It relieves us of the oppressive urgency of the present, the regret of the past, and the fear of the future.

"You will keep him in perfect peace, whose mind is stayed on You, Because he trusts in You. Trust in the Lord forever, for in Yah, the Lord, is everlasting strength." - Isa. 26:3-4.

Prayer is our proper attitude towards the Creator. It is a confession of our limitedness, our inadequacies and our earnest need for guidance and wisdom.

Rev. Franklin Loehr in his book, *The Power of Prayer on Plants,* proves the power of prayer in the growth of plants, from plant seedlings to time of harvest, a difference that can be measured in a laboratory. Plant seeds and seedlings that received prayer grew more rapidly and flourished to a greater extent than those that did not receive prayer. It illustrates how prayer can further improve the quality our lives. Rev. Loehr states that prayer is a form of energy, like sunlight or electricity; and that it is not merely a state of mind.

To experience life more abundantly, continue in the raw vegan diet and practice the other health-related factors that are described not only in this chapter, but throughout this book. Prayer/ meditation, rest and relaxation, exercise, fresh air, sunshine and the raw vegan diet are a powerful combination.

Positive Thinking

Positive thinking greatly assists the healing / rejuvenation process. It is important to believe in what you are doing. That is why a knowledge of foods and nutrition, and of what causes sicknesses and diseases, should come before dietary changes. Have faith in whole plant foods, in yourself and in Nature, and things will turn around in a relatively short time. It is what you are capable of doing now that counts. Put your trust in the efficacy of raw plant foods to heal and rejuvenate the body, and the powers that heal will deliver the victory to you soon.

Next Steps

As more and more fad diets, miracle treatments and supplements become available and attract the attention of millions, so are more and more people throughout the world discovering the health advantages of eating at variance with the customs of the times, and the simple truth that eating natural plant foods leads to good health. They are taking back responsibility for their health and abandoning culturally accepted foods. Truly, these are the lucky ones.

I encourage you to read the books listed in the Bibliography. They have much to offer the novice as well as the long-time student of foods and nutrition. We all like to eat, but it is only when we learn to eat foods that promote health, not destroy it, that our health flourishes. The books provide valuable information and inspiration that will help all seekers of health. They have been a constant source of encouragement to me on my health journey. Take the time to delve into them and you will be glad that you did.

At this very moment, the cells of your body are changing, and the building materials used for that process are the best there are if you are on the raw vegan diet. The advantages of eating raw plant foods are immeasurable, both to us and to our progeny.

In Closing

The raw vegan diet imposes limits on gratifying our desires for certain foods and disproves the culturally imposed belief that supplementation is necessary for heath, but it does not restrict our lives. Rather, it frees us from becoming the slaves of harmful food habits and cravings, and the irrational use of supplements.

The best preparation for tough times ahead is how we deal with the difficulties encountered today. This book has described how to deal with some of the most perplexing and challenging issues that can ever confront any of us. Were we to acknowledge that everything bad that happens to us is an opportunity in disguise, a lesson to be learned for our benefit and a way of strengthening us in some way, then our trials and tribulations would be much easier to bear and we would be better able to see the intended purpose for them.

After being on the raw vegan diet for some time, there may be a tendency to return to one's former ways of eating, even though the dangers of doing so are well known. But even returning to supplements, such as those that contain inorganic minerals as a filler material or as the main ingredient (such as calcium supplements), will likely cause the return of health issues that the diet has thwarted. Fortunately, the body gives us many feedback signals that can be used to keep us on the right track.

However, to retain the great benefits that have been gained, we must keep our distance from commonly consumed foods and substances that cause ill health. An essential part of wisdom is knowing what we cannot adequately handle. By learning about foods and nutrition and becoming more and more familiar with the practices that are described in this book, we gain the wisdom to keep ourselves in health.

We're not likely to get the answers we need to improve our health from conventional medicine practitioners. Conventional medical training allows for little, if any, instruction on how the body heals itself when it is deprived of foods and drinks that do it harm and provided with the foods and drinks it needs for health. In addition, it takes a while for conventional medicine to recognize the merits of treatments that do not employ their approved methods, and even longer to put such treatments into practice. Therefore, each of us must make the difference in our health by solving as many health problems as we can.

We find the answers we are looking for when we dig hard enough for them.

The feelings of exuberance and goodness that result from the eating raw plant foods and combining them properly are the opposite feelings experienced on ordinary diets because of poor nutrition, poor digestion and constipation. The life force properties of raw plant foods make the difference.

By adopting a whole plant food diet, such as the raw vegan diet, sufferers of many of the ill-health conditions of modern times are preparing themselves for a great springtime of health that will affect their lives in extraordinary ways for years to come.

However, the times require vigilance if we wish to maintain the great strides that have been made in the availability of raw fruits and vegetables, and organic plant foods.

We are being thrust into a future that may not be beneficial health-wise for us. We need to keep an eye out for what's ahead, what's around the corner. If raw plant foods (for human consumption) get to be big business, the meat-, grain- and dairy-based interests may feel threatened and apply pressure on the producers and suppliers of these foods. Hopefully, that is a long way off. it seems at least that raw plant foods may never cause a mass exodus away from the Standard American diet.

One of the greatest physicists, Max Planck, said that over the temple of science should be written the words, "Ye must have faith." The great apostle Paul wrote to his new church in Thessalonica, "Prove all things; hold fast that which is good." A scientist says, "Have faith." A saint says "Prove all things." Together, they spell HOPE.

Bibliography

The following books were the major resources used to write this book.

1. T. Colin Campbell, The China Study, 2006.

2. Dr. Michael Greger, How Not To Die, 2015.

3. John Smith, Fruits and Farinacea- The Proper Food of Man, 2015.

4. Russell T. Trall, Scientific Basis of Vegetarianism, 1970.

5. Dr. Caldwell Esselstyn, Jr., Prevent and Reverse Heart Disease, 2007.

6. Jethro Kloss, Back to Eden, 2014.

7. Dr. Ann Wigmore, Be Your Own Doctor, 1982.

8. Dr. Ann Wigmore, Why You Do Not Have to Grow Old, 1985.

9. Dr. Ann Wigmore, The Sprouting Book, 1986.

11. Arnold Ehret, The Mucusless Diet Healing System, 2015.

11. Arnold Ehret, Physical Fitness Through a Superior Diet, Fasting, and Dietetics , 2018.

12. Arnold Ehret, Rational Fasting and Roads to Health and Happiness, 2002.

13. Arnold Ehret, The Cause and Cure of Human Illness, 2001.

14. Teresa Mitchell, My Road to Health, 1987.

15. Norman W. Walker, Colon Health, 2005.

16. Norman W. Walker, Become Younger, 1978.

17. Norman W. Walker, Fresh Vegetable and Fruit Juices, 1978.

18. Norman W. Walker, Diet and Salad Suggestions, 1985.

19. Norman W. Walker, <u>Water Can Undermine Your Health</u>, 1995.

20. Norman W. Walker, <u>The Natural Way to Vibrant Health</u>, 1972.

21. Norman W. Walker, <u>The Vegetarian Guide to Diet and Salad</u>, 1985.

22. Victoria Boutenko, <u>Green for Life</u>, 2005.

23. Victoria Boutenko, <u>12 Steps to Raw Foods</u>, 2005.

24. David Wolfe, <u>The Sunfood Diet Success System</u>, 2008.

25. David Wolfe, <u>Longevity Now: A Comprehensive Approach</u>, 2013.

26. David Wolfe, <u>Superfoods, the Food and Medicine of the Future</u>, 2009.

27. Harvey Diamond, <u>Fit for Life Not Fat for Life</u>, 2003.

28. Harvey Diamond, <u>Living Without Pain</u>, 2007.

29. Dr. D. C. Jarvis, <u>Folk Medicine</u>, 1958.

30. D. C. Jarvis, <u>Arthritis & Folk Medicine</u>, 1960.

31. Robert O. Young and Shelly R. Young, <u>The pH Miracle</u>, 2010.

32. Paul C. and Patricia Bragg, <u>Apple Cider Vinegar, Miracle Health System</u>, 2008.

33. Paul C. and Patricia Bragg, <u>Miracle of Fasting</u>, 2005

34. Dr. Edward Howell, <u>Enzyme Nutrition</u>, 1985.

35. Paul C. and Patricia Bragg, <u>Water, The Shocking Truth That Can Save Your Life</u>, 2004.

36. Professor Spira, <u>Spira Speaks, Dialogs and Essays on The Mucusless Diet Healing System</u>, 2014.

37. Dr. Bernard Jensen, <u>Guide to Diet and Detoxification</u>, 2000.

38. Dr. Bernard Jensen, <u>The Healing Power of Chlorophyll</u>, 1973.

39. Fred S. Hirsch, Internal Cleanliness, 1987.

40. Tonya Zavasta, Beautiful on Raw Uncooked Creations, 2005.

41. Kristina Carrillo-Bucaram, The Fully Raw Diet, 2016.

42. Karyn Calabrese, Soak Your Nuts, 2011.

43. Herbert M. Shelton, Superior Nutrition, 1994.

44. Herbert M. Shelton, Fasting Can Save Your Life, 1978.

45. Herbert M. Shelton, Food Combining Made Easy, 1982.

46. Dr. Russel Blaylock, Excitotoxins, The Taste that Kills, 1997.

47. Joe Alexander, Blatant Raw Foodist Propaganda, 2005.

48. Horst Kornberger, Global Hive: Bee Crisis and Compassionate Ecology, 2012.

49. Annie Payson Call, Power Through Repose, 1905.

50. Steve Meyerowitz, Sprouts, The Miracle Food, 1997.

51. Dr. Henry Lindlahr, Philosophy of Natural Therapeutics, 1975.

52. Dan Georgakas, The Methuselah Factors, 1980.

53. Alexander Leaf, M.D., Youth in Old Age, 1975.

54. Andrew Weil, M.D., Healthy Aging, 2005.

55. Luigi Cornaro, Sure Methods of Attaining a long and Healthful Life, 1660.

56. Luigi Cornaro, The Surest Method of Correcting an Infirm Constitution, 1660.

57. Luigi Cornaro, How to Live 100 Years, or Discourses on the Sober Life, 1660.

58. Dr. Johnny Lovewisdom, Dietetics Vitarianism, 2001.

59. Gabriel Cousens, M.D., Conscious Eating, 2000.

60. Jeffery M. Smith, Genetic Roulette, 2007.

61. F. Batmanghelidj, M.D, Your Body's Many Cries for Water, 2008.

62. Dr. Allen E. Banik, The Choice is Clear, 1989.

63. Robert Morse, N.D., The Detox Miracle Sourcebook, 2004.

64. Arnold Paul De Vries, Therapeutic Fasting, 1958

65. Dr. Kristine Nolfi, M.D., The Miracle of Living Foods, 1981.

66. T. Colin Campbell and Howard Jacobson, Whole: Rethinking the Science of Nutrition, 2014.

67. Wallace D. Wattles, Health Through New Thought and Fasting, 2007.

68. Francoise Wilhelmi de Toledo, MD, and Hubert Hohler, Therapeutic Fasting: The Buchinger Amplius Method, 2018.

69. Edward Hooker Dewey, M.D., The No-Breakfast Plan and the Fasting Cure. 1900.

70. Edward Hooker Dewey, M.D., The True Science of Living. 1894.

71. Upton Sinclair, The Fasting Cure, 1911.

72. Hereward Carrington, Vitality, Fasting and Nutrition, 1908.

73. Paavo O. Airola, N.D., There is a Cure for Arthritis, 1968.

74. Alfred Armand Montapert, The Supreme Philosophy of Man: The Laws of Life, 1977.

75. Edmond Bordeaux Szekely (Translator), The Essene Gospel of Peace, Book One, 1981.

76. Edmond Bordeaux Szekely (Translator), The Essene Gospel of Peace, Book Four, The Teachings of the Elect, 1981.

77. Edmond Bordeaux Szekely (Translator), The Discovery of the Essene Gospel of Peace, 1937.

78. Herbert M. Shelton, Health for the Millions, 1968.

79. O. L. M. Abramowski, Fruitarian Diet and Physical Rejuvenation, 1916.

80. Prof. Arnold Ehret's Mucusless Diet Healing System: Annotated, Revised, and Edited by Prof. Spira, 2015.

81. Sergei and Valya Boutenko, Eating Without Heating, 2002.

82. The Natural Hygiene Handbook, 1996.

83. NIH (National Institutes of Health) Record, April 2015.

84. Rev. Franklin Loehr, The Power of Prayer on Plants, 1959.

85. Victoria Boutenko, Raw & Beyond, 2012.

86. William Meninger, OCSO, The Loving Search for God, 1996.

87. Father Martin Von Cochem, The Four Last Things: Death, Judgement, Hell, Heaven, 2019.

88. The Complete Works of St. John of the Cross, Doctor of the Church, 2010:

89. G. Edmond Griffin, World Without Cancer, 2004.

90. Rich Anderson, Cleanse & Purify Thyself, 2000.

91. Howard F. Lyman, Mad Cowboy, 1998.

92. Brother Lawrence, The Practice of the Presence of God in Modern English, Translated by Marshall Davis, 2013.

93. Eckhart Tolle, The Power of Now, 1999.

94. Stan Shepherd, Raw Veganism, 2018.

95. Stan Shepherd, Stop Sciatica and Spinal Stenosis, 2019.

96. Stan Shepherd, <u>How to Completely Get Rid of Hemorrhoids Naturally: A Permanent Cure</u>, 2019.

97. Stan Shepherd, <u>The Cure for Arthritis</u>, 2020.

About the Author

S. H. Shepherd, 70, has researched and studied the human health field for over 30 years. An engineer by training, he has witnessed the rapid decline of health in this country over the years due to commonly eaten foods. The vital importance of telling others about the many health hazards associated with commonly eaten foods has been the incentive for writing this book.

Biographical:

I grew up in Michigan during the 50's and 60's. I witnessed the fervid race to the moon as well as the initial establishment of the fast food chains. When I was in grade school, my sandwiches were made of boloney or olive loaf slices between two mustard-spread slices of white Wonder Bread. My lunch box included a thermos for milk, but I usually bought a small carton of chocolate milk at the vending machines and a mini-bag of chips or Fritos. I ate what my parents ate and what was advertised on TV. Breakfast was usually Corn Pops, Sugar Pops, Chex, Cheerios, Wheaties, etc., with milk and table sugar. Dinner was often Swanson's TV Dinners. I can't remember seeing a salad during my growing up years except maybe at a restaurant. Dessert was typically ice cream, pie, cake or pudding.

On weekends, breakfast could be bacon and eggs, or sausage and eggs, with white toast and jam or jelly, or pancakes or waffles with butter or margarine and syrup. For road trips, lunch was McDonald's or Burger King hamburgers or cheeseburgers, with fries and a coke or shake. The local Dairy Queen had creamy chocolate cones that weighed about a pound.

A Christian Diet

This gives the reader some idea of the American foodscape at the time I was growing up. Has anything really changed since then?

Had I been raised in a family that practiced a different kind of diet, such as a whole plant food diet, I'm sure I would have learned to eat healthier foods at an early age. That not being the case, I had to learn about foods and nutrition on my own.

Appendices

Appendix I: Berg's Tables

Ragmar Berg's Tables[12] list what foods are acid-binding and acid-forming. As explained in the chapter on "Causes of Disease," these terms are synonymous with mucus-binding and mucus-forming, respectively.

The larger the "plus" or "acid-binding" value, the more the mucus-binder or eliminator the food is. The larger the "minus" or "acid-forming" value, the more the mucus-producer the food is.

According to these tables, meat and grain products are the most acid-forming foods, whereas fruits and vegetables are most acid-binding foods. In other words, meat and grain products are the most mucus-producing foods, whereas fruits and vegetables are the most mucus-eliminating foods.

---

[12] Data taken from the tables published in Arnold Ehret's book, Mucusless Diet Healing System, and the tables available on the Web at the time of this writing.

Name of Food	Plus or Acid-Binding	Minus or Acid-Forming
Flesh		
Meat (Beef)		-38.61
Chicken		-24.32
Ham, Smoked		-6.95
Meat (Beef)		-38.61
Mutton		-20.30
Bacon		-9.90
Ox Tongue		-10.60
Pork		-12.47
Rabbit		-22.36
Veal		-22.95
Fish		
Herring, Salted		-17.35
Oysters	+10.25	
Salmon		-8.32
Shellfish		-19.52
Whitefish		-2.75
Eggs		
Eggs, Whole		-11.61
Eggs, White		-8.27
Eggs, Yolk		-51.83
Milk & Milk Products		
Butter, Cow		-4.33
Buttermilk	+1.31	
Cream	+2.66	
Lard		-4.33
Margarine		-7.31
Milk, Cow	+1.69	
Milk, Goat	+0.65	
Milk, Human	+2.25	
Milk, Sheep	+3.27	
Milk, Skim	+4.89	
Swiss Cheese		-17.49

Name of Food	Plus or Acid-Binding	Minus or Acid-Forming

Grains and Grain Products

Name of Food	Plus or Acid-Binding	Minus or Acid-Forming
Barley		-10.58
Black Bread		-8.54
Cakes (White Flour)		-12.31
Cornmeal		-5.37
Farina		-10.00
Graham Bread		-6.13
Macaroni		-5.11
Oat Flakes		-20.71
Oat Flour		-8.08
Oats		-10.58
Pumpernickel Bread	+4.28	
Quaker Oats		-17.65
Rice, Polished		-17.96
Rice, Unpolished		-3.18
Rye		-11.31
Rye Flour		-0.72
Wheat, Refined		-8.32
Wheat, Whole		-2.66
White Bread		-10.99
Zwieback		-10.41

Vegetables

Name of Food	Plus or Acid-Binding	Minus or Acid-Forming
Asparagus	+1.10	
Artichoke	+4.31	
Cabbages	+4.02	
Cauliflower	+3.09	
Chicory	+2.33	
Dandelion	+17.52	
Dill	+18.36	
Endives	+14.51	
Green Beans	+5.15	
Kohlrabi Root	+5.99	
Milk, Skim	+4.89	
Leeks	+11.00	
Lettuce, Head	+14.12	
Mushrooms	+1.80	

Name of Food	Plus or Acid-Binding	Minus or Acid-Forming
Red Cabbage	+2.20	
Red Onions	+1.09	
Rhubarb	+8.93	
Spinach	+28.01	
String Beans (Fresh)	+8.71	
Watercress	+4.98	

Root Vegetables

Black Radish, with Skin	+39.40	
Celery Roots	+11.31	
Horseradish	+3.06	
Red Beets	+11.33	
Sugar Beets	+9.37	
Sweet Potatoes	+10.31	
White Potatoes	+5.90	
White Turnips	+10.80	
Young Radish	+6.05	

Fruits

Apples	+1.38	
Apricots	+4.79	
Banana	+4.38	
Blackberries	+7.14	
Cherries	+2.57	
Cucumbers	+13.50	
Currants	+4.43	
Dates, Dried	+5.50	
Figs	+27.81	
Grapes	+7.15	
Lemons	+9.90	
Olives	+30.56	
Oranges	+9.61	
Peaches	+5.40	
Pears	+3.26	
Pineapple	+3.59	
Plums	+5.80	
Pomegranates	+4.15	

Name of Food	Plus or Acid-Binding	Minus or Acid-Forming
Prunes	+5.80	
Pumpkins	+0.28	
Raisins	+15.10	
Raspberries	+5.19	
Sour Cherries	+4.33	
Strawberries	+1.76	
Sweet Cherries	+2.66	
Tangerines	+11.77	
Tomatoes	+13.67	
Watermelon	+1.83	

Nuts

Acorns	+13.60	
Almonds		-2.19
Chestnuts		-9.62
Coconut	+4.09	
Hazelnuts		-2.08
Walnuts		-9.22

Legumes

Beans, dried		-9.70
Lentils		-17.80
Peanuts		-16.39
Peas		-3.41
Soy Beans	+26.58	

Drinks, Sweets

Cocoa		-4.79
Chocolate		-8.10
Tea leaves	+53.50	
Coffee	+5.60	

Appendix II: The Dirty Dozen and The Clean Fifteen

Several years ago, the Environmental Working Group (EWG) published lists of fruits and vegetables known as the Dirty Dozen and the Clean Fifteen. These lists indicate foods with the most and least pesticide residues on them based on data compiled by the USDA. The lists are updated annually. They reflect pesticide residues found on foods after they were washed with water.

The Dirty Dozen

The foods highest on this list have the most pesticides on them.

1. Strawberries
2. Apples
3. Nectarines
4. Peaches
5. Celery
6. Grapes
7. Cherries
8. Spinach
9. Tomatoes
10. Sweet bell peppers
11. Cherry tomatoes
12. Cucumbers

According to EWG, buying organic for the twelve fruits and vegetables on this list can reduce our pesticide exposure by at least 90 percent!

The Clean Fifteen

The foods highest on this list have the least pesticides on them.

1. Avocados
2. Sweet corn
3. Pineapples
4. Cabbage
5. Sweet peas (frozen)
6. Onions
7. Asparagus
8. Mangoes
9. Papayas
10. Kiwi
11. Eggplant
12. Honeydew melon
13. Grapefruit
14. Cantaloupe
15. Cauliflower

There is no need to buy organic for the fruits and vegetables on this list, except for cabbage (number 4) and papayas (number 9). For cabbage, according to David Wolfe's book, The Sunfood Diet Success System, non-organic cabbage has large amounts of pesticides are used on it. Papayas are GMO foods and have pesticides on them.

Some types of produce are more prone to containing pesticides residues than others. Avocados, sweet corn and pineapples, for example, are not so prone because of their protective outer layer of skin. Not the same for strawberries and other berries.

Index

Made in the USA
Las Vegas, NV
06 August 2021